Stop Dieting to Finally Lose Weight!

Intuitive Fasting: The Fast Track for Forever Weight Loss

Jannah Adams

© **Copyright 2022 - All rights reserved.**

The content contained within this book may not be reproduced, duplicated or transmitted without direct written permission from the author or the publisher.

Under no circumstances will any blame or legal responsibility be held against the publisher, or author, for any damages, reparation, or monetary loss due to the information contained within this book, either directly or indirectly.

Legal Notice:

This book is copyright protected. It is only for personal use. You cannot amend, distribute, sell, use, quote or paraphrase any part, or the content within this book, without the consent of the author or publisher.

Disclaimer Notice:

Please note the information contained within this document is for educational and entertainment purposes only. All effort has been executed to present accurate, up to date, reliable, complete information. No warranties of any kind are declared or implied. Readers acknowledge that the author is not engaged in the rendering of legal, financial, medical or professional advice. The content within this book has been derived from various sources. Please consult a licensed professional before attempting any techniques outlined in this book.

By reading this document, the reader agrees that under no circumstances is the author responsible for any losses, direct or indirect, that are incurred as a result of the use of the information contained within this document, including, but not limited to, errors, omissions, or inaccuracies.

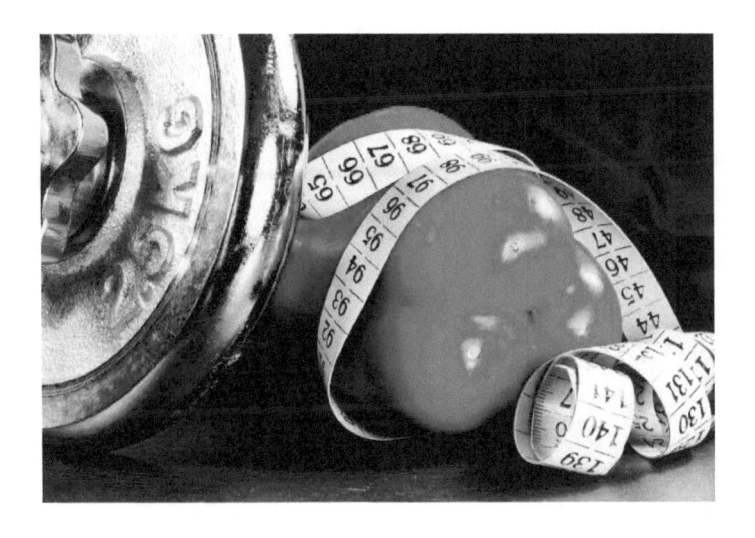

A Special Gift to our Readers!

*Included with your purchase of this book
is our Secrets for incredible weight loss*

This includes:

- Beginner Tips!
- What You Can Eat!
- How to boost your intuitive fasting results!
- Intuitive Fasting Success Stories! What are their ingredients to reach incredible weight loss!

Click the link below and let us know which email address to deliver it to.

www.jannahadams.com

Table of Contents

INTRODUCTION: THE WEIGHT LOSS CHALLENGE 1

CHAPTER 1: WHAT IS INTUITIVE FASTING? 7
   INTUITIVE FASTING: A HISTORY 9
   WHAT HAPPENS WHEN YOU CROSS INTUITIVE EATING WITH
   INTERMITTENT FASTING? 12
   SO WHAT'S ALL THE HYPE ABOUT? 14
   CONCLUSION 15

CHAPTER 2: COMBINING INTUITIVE EATING AND INTERMITTENT FASTING 17
   INTUITIVE EATING 18
      Get Rid of the "Diet Mentality" 20
      Honor the Hunger You Feel 21
      Stop Seeing Food as "the Enemy" 22
      Challenge Your Inner Food Police 22
      Recognize and Respect Your Feelings of Fullness 23
      Discover What Makes You Feel Satisfied 24
      Accept Your Feelings and Cope Without Using Food 24
      Accept, Respect, and Love Your Body 25
      Get Moving and Feel the Difference 26
      Focus On Gentle Nutrition 26
   INTERMITTENT FASTING 28
      16:8 Method 29
      Eat-Stop-Eat 30
      The 5:2 Diet 30
   BRINGING THEM TOGETHER 34
   CONCLUSION 35

CHAPTER 3: THE BIOLOGICAL BENEFITS OF INTERMITTENT FASTING 37

THE EFFECTS OF INTUITIVE EATING 39
   Lower BMI 39
   Lower Risk of Developing Eating Disorders 40
   Improved Interoceptive Awareness 42
THE EFFECTS OF INTERMITTENT FASTING 43
   Production of the Human Growth Hormone Increases 43
   Insulin Sensitivity Improves 44
   Increases the Metabolic Rate 44
   Promotes Cellular Repair 45
   Triggers Gene Expression 46
   Prevents Diseases and Improves Longevity 46
WILL I GET BENEFITS FROM BOTH? 47
CONCLUSION 49

CHAPTER 4: INCREASING MINDFULNESS AND SELF-AWARENESS 51

MINDFUL EATING: HOW THIS CAN HELP YOU TO EAT INTUITIVELY 53
HOW TO EAT MINDFULLY 55
   Reflect on Your Food Issues With Mindfulness 56
   Gradually Get Rid of Unhealthy, Addictive Foods 57
   Start Using Your Senses BEFORE You Eat 57
   Pause Before You Eat 58
   Take a Moment to Appreciate the Food in Front of You .. 59
   Observe Yourself 59
   Tune Into Your Physical Hunger 59
   Eat With Awareness 61
   Pause in the Middle of Your Meal 61
   Practice Mindful Reflection After Your Meal 62
OTHER WAYS TO LISTEN TO YOUR BODY 62
   Stop Watching Those Numbers! 63
   Learn How to Awaken Your Mind-Body Connection 64
   Be Aware of What Your Body Needs Right Now 64
   Find Out What Your Body Needs in the Future 65
CONCLUSION 65

CHAPTER 5: SUPPLEMENTS YOU MAY WISH TO CONSIDER ... 67

EIGHT SUPPLEMENTS YOU NEED 68
   B-Vitamins 68

Magnesium 70
Multivitamins 72
Omega-3 Supplements 73
Probiotics 74
Vitamin C 75
Vitamin D 76
Zinc Supplements 77
CONCLUSION 78

CHAPTER 6: PHASE 1: STARTING INTUITIVE FASTING 79

WHAT IS THE 12:12 FAST? 80
MAKING HEALTHY FOOD CHOICES 82
SAMPLE DAILY ROUTINE 85
INCORPORATING INTUITIVE EATING 87
DOES IT REALLY WORK? 91
CONCLUSION 93

CHAPTER 7: PHASE 2: GETTING THE HANG OF IT 95

WHAT IS THE 16:8 FASTING METHOD? 97
WHAT ARE ITS BENEFITS? 99
HEALTHY FOOD CHOICES 101
TIPS TO HELP FIGHT HUNGER PAINS 104
CONCLUSION 107

CHAPTER 8: PHASE 3: PUSHING TOWARD SUCCESS 109

WHAT IS OMAD? 110
WHAT CAN I EAT? 112
THE BENEFITS OF OMAD 115
ARE THERE ANY RISKS? 119
CONCLUSION 121

CHAPTER 9: PHASE 4: RESET AND RECOVER 123

WHY GO BACK TO THE 12:12 FASTING METHOD? 124
HEALTHY LIFESTYLE TIPS 127
WAYS TO REDUCE INFLAMMATION 131
CONCLUSION 133

CHAPTER 10: STRATEGIES FOR OVERCOMING COMMON FASTING CHALLENGES 135

People Who Shouldn't Fast 136
Nine Potential Side Effects and How to Prevent or Deal With Them 138
    Hunger and Cravings 138
    Malnutrition 140
    Dehydration 141
    Digestive Issues 142
    Bad Breath 143
    Headaches and Lightheadedness 144
    Irritability and Other Mood Changes 146
    Fatigue and Low Energy 147
    Sleep Issues 148
Conclusion 149

CHAPTER 11: SAMPLE RECIPES 151

Greek-Style Chickpea Waffles 152
Whole Wheat Pasta With Turkey Meatballs 155
Savory Fish Cakes With Dipping Sauce 158
Chicken Burrito Bowls 161
Conclusion 165

CONCLUSION: START YOUR WEIGHT LOSS JOURNEY NOW! 167

REFERENCES 170

IMAGE REFERENCES 187

Introduction:

The Weight Loss Challenge

"If you have discipline, drive, and determination... nothing is impossible."—Bailey

These days, there are so many diets and health trends out there that it's impossible to find the right one. Women who want to start living healthier lives try out different diet trends, only to get disappointed when they realize that nothing seems to work.

Does this situation sound familiar?

We've all been there. Feeling like you want to make a change, but also feeling uncertain because you don't know how to do it. When you start a new diet, you are highly motivated. But as the days, weeks, and months go by and you don't see any changes, you end up feeling unhappy and unmotivated. Each time you go through this process, you feel more and more frustrated. And the worst part is, you might end up feeling like you're the only one who is going through such issues.

But you're not.

The truth is, around 95 percent of diets fail (Weiss, n.d.). Not only that, but most people who have successfully lost weight by following a diet have regained the weight they lost in one to five years! Sadly, 35 percent of "occasional dieters"—people who go from one diet to another without ever following through—with time eventually become pathological dieters (Weiss, n.d.). And around a quarter of these eventually develop eating disorders. These are some pretty grim statistics, aren't they? But they do show how so many people all over the world have put in a lot of effort to lose weight and achieve their fitness goals.

Since you are reading this book, it means that you are still looking for a way to lose weight and live a healthier life. Good for you! At some point, we should all make that choice. As someone who has personally struggled through so many challenges in terms of weight loss, I understand the pain and frustration that you feel. We all have those moments of hopelessness. But try not to cling to those. Instead, look out for moments of enlightenment when you decide to do something that will change your life. Right now, you are in one such moment!

Many years ago, I had faced what I felt were endless struggles as I tried to lose weight. I always felt bad about my weight, and it always felt like something that was holding me back. As I tried (and failed) trying different diets, I came to a point where I realized something important. If I wanted to make a change, I needed to learn how to love myself first. Rather than feel frustrated with how I looked, I learned how to accept myself. I stopped going on fad diets for a while because I knew that they weren't working anyway. It wasn't easy, but I gradually learned how to love, appreciate, and be grateful for who I am. When I reached a place where I was happy, I continued my path toward self-improvement.

With a new and positive perspective, I researched first. I didn't jump into the trendiest diet at that time. Instead, I first tried to understand the different types of diets available to me—and that's when I discovered intuitive fasting. I first learned about it after reading an article about Gwyneth Paltrow, the famous actress. She's one of my favorite actresses; so when she has something to say, I'm always interested. According to her, she had also tried various diets and eating patterns over the years. But when she started eating intuitively, she realized that it was the right path for her. She even said that intuitive eating made her feel her best.

In this book, you will learn all about intuitive fasting. This is a type of "road map" to help you train yourself to eat intuitively. The creator of the diet has provided a very clear and simple program that will help you feel good about yourself without having to feel restricted or punished. Basically, you will learn how to listen to your body, your intuition, and yourself. If you have already heard about intuitive eating and intermittent fasting, then understanding this "new diet" will be very easy for you. This is because intuitive fasting combines these diets along with all the benefits they offer.

As a registered dietitian, I have spent over 15 years working within the health and nutrition industry. I now specialize in helping women lose weight effectively—and keeping the weight off for good. While I learned about intuitive fasting, I also developed my own unique plan for weight loss using this wonderful program. Through this unique plan, I have lost 25 pounds! And now, I feel happier and healthier than ever. I even noticed that my energy levels have improved immensely, too. I have also dedicated myself to learning how to make healthy and delicious recipes to help my clients eat more healthily without sacrificing flavor (or satisfaction). Through this book, you will do all of these things and more. In other words, you will learn how to achieve significant weight loss quickly and with minimal effort.

Now, doesn't that sound amazing?

If you are feeling frustrated or defeated right now, you don't have to feel that way for long. I completely understand the difficulties women endure as they try to lose weight along with the expenses that come with trying new diets. It's time to stop the never-ending cycle now. It's time to improve your life.

No matter who you are, what you do, or how much you earn, you will discover what you need within the pages of this book. It's time to pick yourself up once again—and this time, try something that will actually work. At the end of your journey, you won't just lose weight. You will also gain a new perspective on life while learning to love yourself along the way. So if you're ready to explore what intuitive fasting is all about and how to start listening to your body, turn the page and let's begin!

Chapter 1:

What Is Intuitive Fasting?

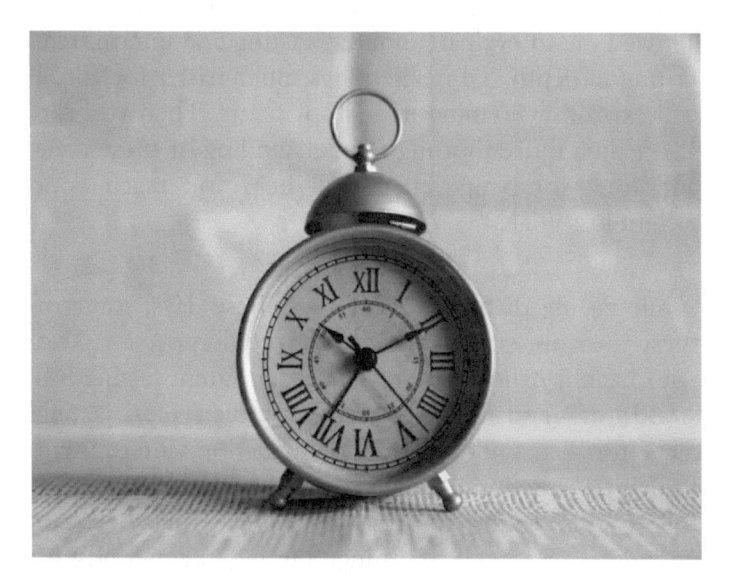

Intuitive fasting is a simple concept, but it's still important to understand all aspects of this diet so that you can follow it safely and correctly. Therefore, we should first discuss the basics of intuitive fasting along with intermittent fasting, which is another beneficial diet that you need to know about. As I have mentioned, I've developed my own unique plan for following intuitive fasting; so you will learn more than the basics. In this chapter, you will discover the following sections:

- Intuitive Fasting: A History

- What Happens When You Cross Intuitive Eating With Intermittent Fasting?

- So What's All the Hype About?

The years of training and experience I possess have allowed me to evaluate intuitive fasting and intermittent fasting in depth. To make things much easier for you, I will explain everything in a simpler way. Then you can also gain a more thorough understanding of these diets and how combining them will help you reach your weight loss goals.

While fasting diets are all the rage these days, some of these diets are either ineffective or could pose a risk to your health. Among these diets, intermittent fasting has stood out—and for good reason. While typical fasting diets focus mainly on caloric restriction, intermittent fasting (IF) focuses on time-restricted eating. When you follow this eating pattern, you will cycle between periods of fasting and eating. During the periods of eating, you have to make sure that you nourish your body and provide it with all of the nutrients it needs to stay healthy. By planning this eating pattern well, you won't have to feel restricted or deprived while following it. The theory behind IF is that humans (along with other animals) have undergone evolutionary physiological adaptations that have allowed them to survive periods of not being able to eat due to scarcity or absence of food. During these periods, our metabolism changes along with how our bodies use energy. Our bodies start using our fat stores for energy, essentially making them efficient fat-burning machines. This is why weight loss is one of the most common benefits of IF. It's also the reason why many people have started following this trendy eating pattern.

But those who cannot sustain IF long-term tend to fall back into their normal eating patterns. When this happens, they could regain the weight they lost along with a few extra pounds. This is where intuitive eating comes in. When you learn how to eat intuitively, you will train yourself to follow healthier eating habits while learning how to endure fasting periods that grow increasingly longer over time. Taking advantage of our evolutionary adaptation that began with our ancestors, and using this along with ancient practices of mindfulness make for a winning combination that will help you achieve your health and weight loss goals!

Intuitive Fasting: A History

The concept of intuitive fasting came from Dr. Will Cole, one of the leading functional medical experts who specializes in the clinical investigation of the factors that cause various chronic diseases. He also consults with people all around the world who suffer from brain problems, digestive disorders, thyroid issues, hormonal dysfunctions, and autoimmune conditions to help them come up with customized health programs that will improve their health.

For a lot of people, the mere idea of only eating one or two meals a day sounds too difficult. This is especially true for people who are used to eating three square meals a day with snacks in between. This has become the norm for a lot of us. We are used to eating every few hours just because there are 'set' meal times—namely breakfast, lunch, and dinner. But the fact is, this isn't the most optimal or natural eating schedule for our bodies. In fact, eating those three regular meals each day can lead to metabolic inflexibility. This, in turn, could lead to other issues like fatigue, inflammation, chronic health issues, and weight gain. For our bodies to function optimally, we need to experience periods of fasting regularly.

This may come as a surprise to you, but it is exactly what Dr. Cole's approach to fasting is all about. Basically, we should learn how to take control of our own hunger. So instead of just following intermittent fasting, you will rely on your intuition to help you discover your instinctive eating patterns. By doing this, you will become more mindful—and thus healthier—in terms of when, how, and even what you eat. Right now, your body is "out of balance" since you are stuck following a pattern that you have learned since you were young. Because of this, it's challenging to rely on your intuition to tell you when you're hungry and when you should eat.

Intuitive fasting is all about learning how to discover metabolic flexibility. It's a combination of intermittent fasting and intuitive eating. Dr. Cole developed a flexible fasting plan that lasts for four weeks. This plan will help you achieve metabolic flexibility so that you can trust your intuition and your body for its ability to function optimally, no matter when you ate your last meal. Each week in this four-week plan allows you to focus on a specific aspect of your health. Once you have completed the four weeks, you will already know how to bring balance back to your hormones, renew your cells, recharge your metabolism, and reset your body.

Dr. Cole's diet is truly a game-changer. Nutritionists, health experts, and—even some of the most popular celebrities such as Gwyneth Paltrow—believe in this diet. It helps you understand the most effective fasting methods while learning how to eat healthily to boost the benefits of the already beneficial diet. Although Dr. Cole's plan is relatively new, the concepts behind it have been around for a very long time. Since you have already tried different diets, it's time to try something that will really help you lose weight while providing other wonderful benefits too!

What Happens When You Cross Intuitive Eating With Intermittent Fasting?

Intuitive fasting is the combination of intuitive eating and intermittent fasting. This combination is supposed to enhance all of the benefits of both diets. Traditionally, intuitive fasting is a program that lasts for four weeks. Within those four weeks, you will cycle through varying fasting windows. For the first week, you will fast for 12 hours every day, which means that your eating window each day would also be 12-hours long. In the second week, you will increase your daily fasting window making it between 14 to 18 hours. In the third week, you will increase your daily fasting window once again. This time, it will be between 20 to 22 hours every other day. And finally, in the fourth week, you will bring back your daily fasting window to 12 hours. At this point, you should have already achieved metabolic flexibility wherein your body can switch from burning carbs to burning fat.

Intuitive fasting is a lot like IF; but the difference is that intuitive fasting encourages you to focus on eating whole, healthy foods like colorful vegetables, fatty fish, olive oil, leafy greens, nuts, seeds, and more. It is akin to following a meal plan that's similar to the ketogenic diet wherein you can cycle between high-carb and low-carb days. This will reduce your risk of experiencing the common adverse side effects of a 'true' keto diet.

The great thing about this diet is that you can use whatever dieting method you would like while following it. Since you will be fasting every day, you will naturally lose weight since you will eat fewer calories daily throughout the four weeks when you will be following this program. Of course, you shouldn't force yourself to eat excessively during your eating windows. If you do this, you won't end up losing weight. Instead, you should try to eat normally during your eating windows; and you can do this by tuning into your body and awakening your natural intuition.

While intuitive fasting is very effective, the 'traditional' intuitive fasting diet isn't necessarily suitable for everyone. If you break the diet down, intuitive eating works well for those who have experience in caloric restriction and calorie tracking. They already know how these processes work, and so they can adjust to intuitive fasting smoothly. Intermittent fasting, on the other hand, works well for those who have already tried fasting in the past.

Either way, you might end up developing some type of fear around food. Fortunately, this guide will help you create a more realistic plan that will help you focus on wellness while learning how to listen to your body. Instead of just following a plan, you will take a sort of journey to self-discovery that will ultimately lead to you achieving your weight loss goals. So you don't have to feel intimidated. We are just at the beginning. Right now, you are still in the process of understanding the basic foundations of this diet so that you can start creating your own plan later on.

So What's All the Hype About?

If you haven't heard about intuitive fasting yet, it's just a matter of time. This is an up-and-coming diet that will potentially become the "new way" of losing weight that everyone will want to try. And the fact that someone as famous (in Hollywood and in the world of health and fitness) as Gwyneth Paltrow has already started following this diet already says a lot. According to Gwyneth, she tried following IF after getting infected with COVID-19. Because of the illness, she experienced some long-term side effects including inflammation, fatigue, and brain fog. When IF didn't work (and nothing else did), her health advisor Dr. Will Cole suggested that she follow intuitive fasting.

Although this program isn't specifically designed to treat diseases, the combination of intuitive eating and IF brings many benefits that can help improve various conditions. At the end of the program, Gwyneth discovered that she developed healthy eating habits naturally without feeling like she was forced into the diet. As the founder of Goop, the wellness and lifestyle brand and company, it's really impressive to discover that someone as passionate about health and wellness would follow this diet. Not only that, but she actually experienced firsthand how it changed her life for the better!

As someone interested in following this diet (or a simpler, guided version of it), you will learn some very important things. You will learn how to listen to your body, eat what feels right, and experience all of the good effects in the process. Before writing this book, I tried the diet too. True enough, I experienced the many benefits of intuitive fasting. And if someone like Gwyneth Paltrow—with all of her knowledge and experience about health—is raving about it, too, then intuitive eating must be worth trying!

Conclusion

In this chapter, you have learned all the basics of intuitive fasting. As you now know, it's not like many other diets that end up making you feel too restricted or deprived. It is an eating pattern that will teach and encourage you to develop healthier eating habits while being more aware of the foods you eat as well. Since it was developed, intuitive fasting has proven effective time and time again. When I started following it, I also noticed that the program helped me lose weight.

While following the program, I realized that it might be a bit challenging—especially for those who don't have enough experience. This is why I decided to make some modifications to it. But before we go into the actual process of following this diet, you must first gain a better understanding of what intuitive eating and intermittent fasting are all about. Knowing these two concepts will help you understand why the combination works wonders and how you can make this program work for you. So keep reading!

Chapter 2:

Combining Intuitive Eating and Intermittent Fasting

Back in the year 1995, the term "intuitive eating" was coined as it was used as the title of a book written by Elyse Resch and Evelyn Tribole. But the actual concept of this approach to eating has been around longer. Back in 1978, Susie Orbach published a book entitled Fat is a Feminist Issue, where she used the concept of intuitive eating (although the actual term wasn't used yet). And in 1982, Geneen Roth also used the same concept as she wrote books about emotional eating.

In 1973, Thelma Wayler founded a Vermont-based weight management program, which was based on the concept of intuitive eating. She developed the program based on the principle that personal care and lifestyle changes are more important and effective since diets don't really work. When you think about it, intuitive eating is based on the same principle. In order to achieve long-term health, you need to learn how to listen to your body instead of allowing yourself to follow a strict schedule or diet wherein you eat even though you don't even feel hungry!

In this chapter, you will learn all about intuitive eating and intermittent fasting—the two foundations of the intuitive fasting diet. You will also discover the benefits of each eating approach and how you can combine them to create your own intuitive fasting plan. This chapter contains the following sections:

- Intuitive Eating

- Intermittent Fasting

- Bringing Them Together

It's time to end the vicious cycle of starting new diets, not being able to follow through, then feeling defeated and frustrated. Now, it's time to learn about two of the most successful diets out there and how putting them together will help you lose weight while bringing other wonderful benefits to your life. As someone who has successfully achieved my health and weight loss goals through intuitive fasting, I am here to tell you that you can do it too. With the right guidance and self-motivation, you can have your own success story to tell in the future!

Intuitive Eating

Intuitive eating is more of an eating style than a diet. It encourages you to adopt a healthier attitude toward your body image and the food you eat. The basic idea behind intuitive eating is to eat whenever you feel hungry and stop eating when you feel full. Eating this way should be an intuitive process. However, because of the "usual timings" we follow (breakfast, lunch, dinner, and snack times), we seldom rely on our intuition when we are eating.

If you keep trying to follow different kinds of diets, it will be very difficult for you to learn how to eat intuitively. Rather than listening to and trusting your body and its natural intuition, you will only focus on the food you eat and the food you are depriving yourself of. But eating intuitively is all about learning how to trust your body. By doing this, you will be able to differentiate the two types of hunger that we can feel:

- **Physical Hunger**

This refers to the biological urge you feel when your body is running out of nutrients and it's time for you to replenish your stores. Physical hunger comes gradually and over time; you will experience various hunger signals such as irritability, fatigue, or a growling stomach. When you nourish yourself by eating food, your physical hunger will be satisfied.

- **Emotional Hunger**

This refers to the urge to eat that comes from some kind of emotional need. Strong emotions like loneliness, sadness, or even boredom can create food cravings which then make you feel like you are hungry.

Often, you can crave comfort foods when you feel emotional hunger. If you give in to this hunger, there is a good chance that you would overeat. When you're done, you can often feel negative emotions like self-hatred and guilt.

Intuitive eating focuses on physical hunger. Since you will learn how to listen to your body, you will also learn how to be aware of your body's natural hunger signals. To become an intuitive eater, you need to understand the 10 principles behind this eating style:

Get Rid of the "Diet Mentality"

The "diet mentality" refers to the idea that there is one diet out there that will help you reach your health and fitness goals. One diet that will magically work for you after you have tried and failed at so many others. Intuitive eating isn't like that. In fact, it's considered the "anti-diet" because you won't have to follow strict rules just to lose weight or achieve whatever results you are expecting. Although some diets may help you lose weight, they won't guarantee that you will keep that weight off in the long run. If you discover that the diet is too challenging, it doesn't seem to be working, or you just can't keep up with it, you might just give up. Then you'll find yourself looking for another diet to try. Unfortunately, this is when you get stuck in a never-ending cycle of diets that make you feel bad about yourself over and over again. Also, if you follow diets that are too restrictive, you might end up depriving your body of the nutrients it needs to function optimally. And for a lot of people, dieting leads to eating disorders, which are much more difficult to deal with.

So you should reject this diet mentality now. Get rid of any books or resources you have that offer false (and often impossible) hopes of quickly losing weight forever. You don't have to try all diet trends just because they are very popular. This culture has become very damaging, especially for people who want to lose weight, keep the weight off, and remain healthy. Instead, focus on learning healthier habits by listening to your body and changing the habits you have now. By doing this, you will open yourself up to the possibility of learning how to eat intuitively.

Honor the Hunger You Feel

Hunger isn't something you should dread. It isn't bad and you shouldn't consider hunger as "the enemy." Many people feel like they cannot lose weight because they either eat too much or eat too often, all because they "feel hungry." But remember that there are two types of hunger: physical and emotional. If you feel the latter and you always give in to your cravings, then you will find it very difficult to lose weight. Before you reach for a bag of chips or a bowl of ice cream, try self-reflecting. Ask yourself if you really feel hungry or if you're just feeling some strong emotions and you want to use food to cope. If it's the latter, try to find something more productive to do.

As for satisfying physical hunger, you must first learn how to recognize the early signs. Then you can nourish your body with the right foods so you will feel satisfied right away. If you are already feeling hungry, eat something. Allowing yourself to get excessively hungry will only lead to overeating. To become more intuitive, know the signs of physical hunger and be more aware when you are feeling them. This will help you become more in tune with your body so that you won't have to feel bad whenever you feel hungry.

Stop Seeing Food as "the Enemy"

As with hunger, food isn't the enemy either. Food nourishes you. Food will help you become healthy and strong. It's time to get rid of the "food rules" you have learned from various diets so that you can start anew. Allow yourself to eat what you want when you feel hungry. Restricting yourself from eating a certain type of food will only increase your cravings. And when you can't stand it anymore, you will end up binging on the food you keep trying to avoid. Get rid of the idea of "forbidden food" so that you won't always feel guilty after eating.

Challenge Your Inner Food Police

After convincing yourself that hunger and food aren't your enemies, work on calming your internal "food police" as well. If you have been following various diets in your attempt to lose weight, you would have developed an inner food police that always dictates what is bad for you, what is good for you, what you should eat, and what you shouldn't eat. When you feel hungry and you spot some food, this food police starts telling you what you should or shouldn't do. Unfortunately, this usually comes with guilt-provoking thoughts, negative ideas, and words that make you feel hopeless. It's time to get rid of your food police as you focus more on learning how to listen to your body and your natural intuition.

Recognize and Respect Your Feelings of Fullness

When it's finally time to eat, you should still continue listening to your body. Just as your body will naturally tell you that you are hungry, it will also tell you when you are full. While eating, try to observe the signals that indicate that you are full and satisfied. One of the best ways to do this is to slow down while eating. Try to observe how the food tastes, how it feels in your mouth while you chew, and how you are feeling after swallowing each mouthful. It's also a good idea to pause once in a while to savor your meal while checking if you are still hungry or if you are already full. If you feel the latter, then you know that it's time to stop.

Discover What Makes You Feel Satisfied

As you are trying to get rid of the negativities you have about food and eating, you should also start looking at the positive side. While allowing yourself to eat different kinds of foods, try to observe what types of foods make you feel satisfied. Doing this will make eating a more enjoyable experience for you. If you eat foods that you like, you will always feel satisfied at the end of a meal. And if you are able to listen to your body when it tells you that you are full, the chances of overeating or binging will decrease dramatically.

Accept Your Feelings and Cope Without Using Food

Another way to awaken your natural intuition is by learning how to cope with your feelings. First, you need to recognize, accept, and honor your feelings. Doing this allows you to cope with them instead of turning to food all the time. For instance, when you feel bored, you can find something interesting to do. When you feel angry, do something that will calm you down. By honoring your feelings, you will eventually get rid of your emotional eating habits. Then you can focus on recognizing your physical hunger and working to satisfy it through food.

Accept, Respect, and Love Your Body

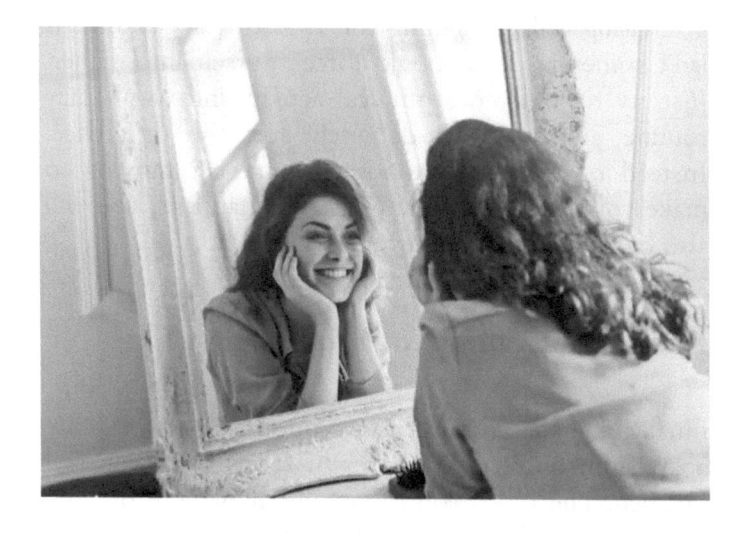

One of the biggest reasons why you end up getting frustrated when diets don't work is because you feel unsatisfied with your body. Unfortunately, such feelings could hinder you from learning how to eat intuitively. Although it's easier said than done, you need to start learning how to accept, respect, and love your body. Remember that your body has given you so much and it continues to work to keep you alive. If you have negative feelings toward your body, these could cloud your natural intuition. So give yourself a break and start focusing on self-love!

Get Moving and Feel the Difference

Exercising isn't something you should feel afraid of. It isn't something you should force yourself into, either. Just try to add more physical activity into your daily routine and you will definitely feel the difference. Instead of exercising to lose weight, get moving to make yourself feel better. When this happens, you will also become more in tune with your body.

Focus On Gentle Nutrition

Finally, you should also focus on nourishing your body apart from finding what types of foods make you feel satisfied. The foods you eat should allow you to enjoy your meals and make your body feel good, too. You don't have to change your diet drastically. Make it a process where you rediscover different foods until you are able to determine which foods nourish you the most, while also making you feel happy and satisfied after you eat.

All of these principles will help you tune in to the physical sensations you feel within your body, while getting rid of any hindrances or obstacles that could weaken your intuition. If you can follow these core principles, then you can truly understand and learn what intuitive eating is all about. This, in turn, will allow you to experience the many benefits of intuitive eating.

This eating approach offers both mental and physical benefits. Mentally, you will develop a more positive body image if you are able to intuitively focus on your physical hunger while giving in to your emotional hunger less and less. And when you see that you are shedding those stubborn excess pounds, you will feel a lot happier, too. In terms of physical benefits, learning how to accurately recognize your body's signals will help you to avoid—or even overcome—any eating disorders, thus improving your overall health. To eat intuitively is simple; apart from the 10 principles, here are some things to keep in mind:

- Pay attention to your existing food habits so that you can change the bad ones and keep the good ones.

- Stop labeling foods as good or bad.

- Before you eat, take a moment to reflect on why you want to eat.

- Learn how to recognize and listen to your body's hunger cues.

- Try some mindfulness techniques to help you overcome emotional eating.

By keeping all of these in mind, you will be able to eat intuitively. And if you can do this, you can also start incorporating intermittent fasting into this eating pattern to create the winning eating approach that you are striving for.

Intermittent Fasting

Intermittent fasting (IF) is not really a diet. It is an eating plan wherein you regularly cycle between periods of fasting and periods of eating. Because of its popularity, a lot of research and studies have been conducted about IF and most of them agree that it is a powerful weight-loss tool. While diets focus on what you should eat, IF focuses on when you should eat.

When you follow IF, you will only eat during specific times each day. The great thing about this eating approach is that you get to set your fasting and eating schedules (IF methods), which means that you can start to slowly allow your body to adjust to fasting. The idea behind IF is that fasting for a certain number of hours per day, or only eating a single meal one or two times each week, will force your body into a metabolic state known as ketosis. Once your body is in ketosis, it starts burning fat for fuel instead of glucose. This is the main reason why intermittent fasting is very effective at promoting weight loss.

When you think about it, fasting has always been a part of our lives. Our ancient ancestors only relied on the foods that they hunted or foraged for. When they couldn't hunt anything and foraging didn't prove productive either, they had no choice but to skip meals. These days, food is readily available, which is why we have gotten used to eating throughout the day. But we don't have to do this. Because of the challenges our ancestors encountered that forced them to fast for hours or days, our bodies have evolved to survive this way of eating. There are several IF methods you can follow, the most common of which are:

16:8 Method

Also known as the Leangains protocol, this method involves eating for 8 hours and then fasting for 16 hours each day. For instance, if you are a morning person, you can start your eating window at 7:00 a.m. wherein you would eat your first meal of the day. For 8 hours, you can eat food whenever you feel hungry. But you must have your last meal before 3:00 p.m. This is when your fasting window begins.

When your fasting window starts, you cannot eat any solid foods or drink any beverages with calories like smoothies or sweetened drinks. But you can keep yourself hydrated by drinking water, plain tea, or plain coffee. This fasting method is a common choice for beginners, since it is fairly easy compared to the other IF methods. When you think about it, the 8 hours you spend sleeping already count as half of your fasting window. So you would only have to get used to not eating anything for the other 8 hours.

If this is your first time trying a fast, you don't have to follow this method every day. You can try it out for a few days each week first, and do this for about 2 weeks. For the next 2 weeks, you can increase the number of days, then keep doing this until you are able to follow this IF method every day.

Eat-Stop-Eat

This involves choosing 2 days in a week where you would fast for 24 hours. For instance, if you choose to fast from 8:00 p.m. on Tuesday, then your fasting window would then last until 8:00 p.m. on Wednesday (the next day). It's best to choose days that are not too close to each other so that you won't feel too overwhelmed with the 24-hour fasting windows. Also, it's not recommended to start with this IF method if you're a beginner, as your body might get shocked if you suddenly try fasting for an entire day without any prior practice.

The 5:2 Diet

This method is similar to the eat-stop-eat method, since you will eat normally for 5 days each week and then fast for the other 2 days, but the difference is that you won't fast completely on your 2 fasting days. Instead, on the 2 nonconsecutive fasting days, you would only eat between 500 to 600 calories throughout the day. This could come in the form of a single meal or several small meals throughout the day. For the other 5 days, you would follow your 'regular' diet. Since you won't fast completely, this could be another option for you if this is your first time following IF.

There are more intense IF methods wherein the fasting periods are either longer or more frequent. But as a beginner, such methods aren't recommended. If you're not used to fasting and you rush into IF, your body might end up storing more fat instead of burning it because it feels like it is being starved. Also, it's important to check with your doctor first before you begin an IF method—especially if you suffer from some type of medical condition or if you are taking medications.

The reason why IF has become so popular is that it offers so many benefits. Let's go through these benefits now before we try combining this eating approach with intuitive eating:

- **Weight Loss**

Weight loss is the most evident benefit of IF, and it's also one of the main reasons why people choose to follow IF. Since you will be fasting for regular amounts of time, you will also be eating fewer meals. When following IF, you shouldn't try to compensate for all of the food you didn't eat while fasting by overeating during your eating windows. If you do this, then you probably won't lose weight. But if you eat normally during your eating windows or if you are able to eat intuitively (only when you are physically hungry), then you will definitely start shedding those stubborn excess pounds.

- **Reduced Insulin Resistance**

This is a very important benefit as it will protect you against type-2 diabetes. By fasting, your insulin levels will go down. When this happens, the fat stores in your body become more accessible, which then allows your body to burn those fat stores to power your body's processes.

- **Reduced Inflammation**

IF can also help reduce the markers of inflammation in the body. This is another significant benefit, since inflammation can contribute to the development of various chronic diseases.

- **Improved Heart Health**

This eating approach reduces the levels of LDL cholesterol, which is considered "bad cholesterol." It also increases the levels of HDL cholesterol, or "good cholesterol." Both of these effects will improve your cardiovascular health.

- **Cancer Prevention**

Another potential benefit of IF is that it can help reduce the risk of cancer. Although there isn't a lot of research that supports this claim, existing research shows promising results. This eating approach can also help enhance the effects of chemotherapy treatments.

- **Improved Brain Health**

IF increases the production of brain-derived neurotrophic factor (BDNF) that promotes the growth of new cells in the brain. This, in turn, can help reduce the risk of brain-related diseases like Parkinson's and Alzheimer's.

- **Anti-aging Benefits**

Studies have shown that IF can extend life span thanks to its anti-aging benefits. This comes from effects like cellular repair and gene expression. Fasting also stimulates life-extending mechanisms in the body through caloric restriction. Even though you don't have to starve or deprive yourself, fasting could still give you a longer life.

- **A Simpler and Healthier Lifestyle**

Finally, IF makes your life simpler. Since you will only eat at certain times of the day, you don't have to plan all of your meals throughout the day. And if you combine this with intuitive eating, your life will become even simpler as you will only eat whenever you feel hungry!

Bringing Them Together

Now that you understand what intuitive eating and intermittent fasting are all about, it's time to start putting them together. I personally had followed the intuitive fasting program, and it helped me lose weight. Over the years, I have developed my own tips and techniques for following this program and I have used these to help my clients. I have witnessed astonishing transformations in my clients; but the ones who had the most significant results were following IF, intuitive eating, or a combination of the two.

On its own, intuitive eating offers both mental and physical benefits. Aside from losing weight, you will also learn how to accept and love yourself, which will make it easier for you to convince yourself to learn and maintain healthier habits. Intermittent fasting also comes with its own benefits, weight loss being the most common one. When you think about it, putting these eating approaches together means that you would be combining their benefits too, right?

Although there is limited research that shows the effects of combining intuitive eating and IF, there is the potential to reap the benefits of both eating approaches if you do them in conjunction with each other. As someone who has tried both diets separately and together, I can tell you that this is definitely a possibility to look forward to. Of course, there is much more to learn about this. So keep reading!

Conclusion

In this chapter, you learned the fundamentals of intuitive eating and intermittent fasting. To summarize, intuitive eating involves learning how to listen to your body's natural hunger signals while also learning how to differentiate physical hunger from emotional hunger. Intermittent fasting, on the other hand, is a unique eating approach wherein you cycle between periods of fasting and periods of eating.

Both intuitive eating and intermittent fasting have their own benefits. And when you combine them together, you can potentially create a new way of eating that allows you to enjoy the benefits of both approaches to eating. Now that you have gained a better understanding of the core concepts of intuitive fasting, you should have a clearer idea of why this program works so well. Although you have been frustrated in the past by following different diets that don't really work, you can now focus on something that will help you lose weight in the long run. To help you understand this even further, let's take a look at the biological side of things, which you will discover in the next chapter.

Chapter 3:

The Biological Benefits of Intermittent Fasting

Whether you will start following intuitive eating, intermittent fasting, or you will combine these two approaches right away, the effects you will experience will happen within your body. To help you understand these changes, we need to focus on the biological processes that happen in your body along with the physical consequences that occur because of intuitive eating and intermittent fasting. In this chapter, you will learn:

- the effects of intermittent fasting
- the effects of intuitive eating

We will also answer the question, "Will combining them mean that you will get the benefits of both?"

As I followed these diets myself, I researched more about them. During my studying and training to become a dietitian, I had also learned a lot about the human body and how it is affected by nutrition. All of these experiences and knowledge have allowed me to help my clients lose weight successfully and reach their health goals.

In order to successfully lose weight, you must first understand your metabolism. This refers to the chemical reactions that occur in the cells of the body wherein food is converted to energy. Around 70 percent of your total caloric intake is converted into energy that your body needs to stay alive. From breathing to generating heat, producing new cells, releasing hormones, and everything in between, your body needs enough food to keep you going. The other 20 percent of the food you eat is converted into energy for more intense physical activities like exercising, walking from one place to another, doing your chores, and more. And the last 10 percent is needed by your body to digest the food you eat at every meal.

If you want to lose weight, you shouldn't just starve yourself. Doing this will mess with your metabolism. Often, you would start feeling weak because your body isn't getting enough food to convert into energy. This causes your metabolism to slow down, thus causing your body to start storing fat to keep you going.

This is just one example of a biological process you need to understand so that you can lose weight in a healthy and sustainable way. In this chapter, I will share the most significant research and studies I have come across while incorporating this information with the two eating approaches we are focusing on. So, let's begin!

The Effects of Intuitive Eating

Intuitive eating is a wonderful eating approach, as it helps you become more aware of your body and your natural instincts. The results of a study revealed that this eating approach is more effective, healthier, and natural compared to other strategies for weight-loss (Denny, et al., 2013). Instead of having to follow strict rules, you will learn how to recognize your physical hunger so that you can satisfy it by eating healthy food. As you start following your intuitive eating journey, it will affect your body in different ways.

Lower BMI

Body mass index (BMI) refers to the measure of a person's body fat based on their weight and height. BMI applies to adult women and men, and there are four categories you could belong to, namely:

- underweight if your BMI is less than 18.5

- normal weight if your BMI ranges between 18.5 and 24.9

- overweight if your BMI ranges between 25 and 29.9

- obese if your BMI is equal to or greater than 30

If you want to determine your BMI, you can use online BMI calculators. You can also visit your doctor for a more accurate measurement. If you discover that your BMI falls under the overweight or obese categories, then intuitive eating can help you lower this. Once you reach your healthy weight, you can continue following your intuition and eating healthily.

Lower Risk of Developing Eating Disorders

One of the biggest risks of following diets, especially strict ones, is developing an eating disorder. When you focus too much on the foods you should eat and how much you should be eating, you could end up feeling deprived. And when you allow yourself to eat what you want, this usually comes with negative feelings like guilt, shame, and frustration. Unfortunately, if this keeps happening, you could end up going down a road that leads to disordered eating.

But when it comes to intuitive eating, there is very little risk of this happening. If you go back to the core principles of intuitive eating, you will notice that they encourage you to adopt a more positive perspective and mindset in terms of food, eating, and accepting yourself. Many studies have been conducted about intuitive eating and disordered eating, and they have all shown promising results. For example, in one study, the researchers discovered that intuitive eating's mindfulness aspect can possibly help to prevent maladaptive dietary restraint, a condition which could cause disordered eating (Anderson et al., 2015). All the while, you can still lose weight and maintain a healthy weight once you have reached your goal. In another study, intuitive eating's mindfulness aspect has proven to also be very helpful in preventing emotional eating and binge eating (Warren, J. M. et al., 2017). These are two significant factors that, if not prevented, could contribute to the development of eating disorders.

In addition, another study has revealed that intuitive eating does really affect eating behaviors in a positive way (Van Dyke & Drinkwater, 2013). In this study, the researchers also noticed improvements in physical health, psychological health, and weight loss. A study conducted more recently has also revealed how this approach to eating can reduce the risk of body dissatisfaction, low self-esteem, depressive symptoms, binge eating, and other extreme behaviors that are associated with weight control (Hazzard et al., 2020). In addition, a fairly recent study examined the specific effects of intuitive eating related to maladaptive eating behaviors (Kerin et al., 2019). This study also showed positive results as the participants had adapted positive behaviors, motivations, and beliefs thanks to the unique eating approach.

These are just some examples that showcase the positive effects of intuitive eating in terms of avoiding disordered eating. Whether you have a history of disordered eating or you are currently struggling with such an issue, intuitive eating can be very beneficial for you.

Improved Interoceptive Awareness

Introceptive awareness refers to your ability to appropriately recognize, identify, accept, and respond to the patterns of your internal signals. In other words, it's your ability to tune into the natural signals of your body. As you already know, this is something that you will learn through intuitive eating. One study has revealed that the use of effective emotional regulation has to involve a sound relationship within oneself, which means that there should be effective communication that flows between the body, feelings, and mind (Price & Hooven, 2018). This same study has shown that there are strong links between introceptive awareness and emotional regulation. This means that if you don't have introceptive awareness, it will be very difficult for you to master emotional regulation.

Since intuitive eating encourages you to change your mindset for it to become more positive, this can help improve your introceptive awareness. Although this won't happen overnight, each step you take toward following this eating approach can help you become more accepting and aware of your thoughts, feelings, and even your physical sensations.

The Effects of Intermittent Fasting

While intermittent fasting is a relatively new concept compared to other diets, the concept behind IF—fasting—has been around since the time of our ancestors. At its core, intermittent fasting encourages you to fast for certain amounts of time each day or for a certain number of days each week. IF has proven to be so effective that many studies have been conducted about it. For example, one study has shown the important role IF plays in the body's different cellular responses (Longo & Mattson, 2014). This is a very important benefit as it offers many positive effects on the body.

Production of the Human Growth Hormone Increases

The production of the human growth hormone (HGH) occurs in the brain, specifically in the hypothalamus. But it is secreted into the bloodstream so that it reaches the different tissues in the body. This hormone is primarily involved in metabolism and growth, which is why growing children and teenagers have high levels of HGH. When you reach adulthood, your HGH hormone levels tend to decrease. But when you fast intermittently, your HGH levels increase significantly. When this happens, you will experience benefits like muscle gain, fat loss, and more. This hormone also plays a role in the metabolism of fat, sugar regulation, cellular regeneration, and bone growth. It can even improve heart functions.

Insulin Sensitivity Improves

Insulin is a type of hormone produced by the pancreas, and it regulates the glucose levels in your bloodstream. This hormone is also responsible for storing glucose in your fat, muscles, and liver. Another function of insulin is the regulation of protein, fat, and carbohydrates in the body. Whenever you eat, this causes an elevation in your blood glucose levels. This, in turn, would stimulate your pancreas to release insulin. But if your insulin sensitivity isn't functioning well, your pancreas won't function well, either. This would cause instabilities or fluctuations in your blood glucose levels, and is one of the main factors that causes diabetes. The good news is, your insulin sensitivity will improve through intermittent fasting. Fasting gives your body time to break down the foods you eat and either utilize or store nutrients properly. This is one of the reasons why IF is recommended for the prevention or management of type-2 diabetes.

Increases the Metabolic Rate

Metabolism is an automatic process that occurs within the body. But your metabolic rate depends on various factors, and fasting is one of those factors. The results of one study showed that your metabolic rate can increase by as much as 14 percent with fasting (Zauner et al., 2000). This is a significant benefit, especially if you want to lose weight. Other factors that affect metabolism are your physical activity levels along with the involuntary physical activities your body does, or the automatic processes that happen naturally such as digestion and breathing.

Promotes Cellular Repair

Fasting also promotes cellular repair along with a process known as autophagy. Autophagy is your body's way of getting rid of damaged, dead, and old cells in order to produce new cells that are much healthier. This process is extremely beneficial to your health, since it helps rejuvenate your body in different ways. Autophagy is also considered a self-preservation mechanism as it uses the damaged and dysfunctional cells to repair, clean, and create new cells. This, in turn, allows your body to function optimally.

Autophagy is also beneficial in terms of anti-aging. Since your body will be producing new cells and repairing old ones, it could help protect you while increasing your lifestyle as well. The great thing about autophagy is that it also allows your body to use cellular material for other necessary bodily processes, too.

Triggers Gene Expression

One study revealed that various metabolic and adaptive hormonal responses in the body are triggered by fasting, and these responses can help improve overall health (Tunstall et al., 2002). One such process is gene expression—this is a process that involves the creation of molecules, proteins, and other end products by using the information found in the genes. In other words, this process is the basis of the development and differentiation of cells. It also allows cells to adapt to different conditions effectively. Fasting triggers this process, which then ensures that your body works smoothly and optimally each day.

Prevents Diseases and Improves Longevity

With all the benefits IF has to offer, it can also protect your body against diseases, which thereby improves your longevity. Researchers discovered in one study that fasting can help slow down the growth of tumors, and that it can also enhance the effects of certain systemic agents and chemotherapy drugs that are used in the treatment of different types of cancer (Zhu et al., 2013). This is just one example of how fasting can help protect you from one of the most devastating diseases in existence. In yet another study, it was discovered by researchers that IF can help improve and promote the nervous system's health (Martin et al., 2006). This is a significant benefit, especially since it can help prevent diseases like Parkinson's and Alzheimer's. Having a healthy nervous system is essential to overall health and longevity. Having a healthy body that's free of diseases also improves your longevity. And both of these are potential benefits of intermittent fasting.

Will I Get Benefits From Both?

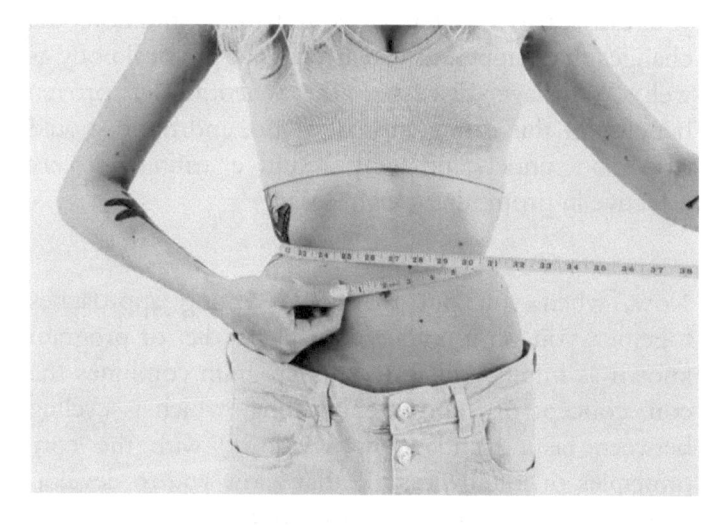

As you can see, both intuitive eating and intermittent fasting cause several good changes within your body. Intermittent fasting is one of the few diet trends that is actually supported by science. Because of its popularity, it has been the focus of several studies, which have provided promising results time and again. Although many of these studies were conducted on animals, the anecdotal evidence from countless people all over the world who have tried and succeeded with IF strengthens these claims. Even nutritionists, dietitians, and health experts agree that this is one of the best diets that promote weight loss while providing other health benefits, too.

Intuitive eating is another eating approach that offers some wonderful benefits while stimulating some significant changes within your body. While intuitive eating focuses more on your mental health and how you can learn to listen to your natural intuition, the changes that happen to you affect your physical body as well. We have discussed the scientifically proven benefits of this eating approach, too, and these should help you understand why intuitive eating is very effective in promoting weight loss.

Now, when you put these two eating approaches together, you get a unique and special diet or program known as intuitive fasting. This program combines the core concept of intermittent fasting (which is cycling between fasting and eating windows) with the core principles of intuitive eating that allow you to develop awareness and attention to your body so that you can always satisfy your physical hunger without giving in to emotional eating. If you can stick with this program, you could enjoy some benefits like:

- an improvement in insulin sensitivity along with lowered levels of fasting glucose

- an increase in HDL or 'good' cholesterol levels and a decrease in your LDL or 'bad' cholesterol levels
- an improvement in your body's fatty acid metabolism and liver protein profiles
- a longer lifespan

You may have noticed that these are the same benefits you can get from IF and intuitive eating. Since you will combine the basic ideas of both diets to come up with a new program that works for you, you can also enjoy the benefits of both eating approaches along the way.

Conclusion

By understanding the physiological benefits of intuitive fasting (the combination of IF and intuitive eating), you will gain a better understanding of why this program works so well as a weight-loss tool. In this chapter, you learned all about the effects of intuitive eating on your body along with the effects of intermittent fasting on your body, too. We also discussed the possibility of gaining the benefits of both eating methods if you combine them into one simple and effective program, known as intuitive fasting. The next step is to prepare yourself for the journey ahead. And you can do this by learning all about mindfulness, which is a big part of intuitive fasting.

Chapter 4:

Increasing Mindfulness and Self-Awareness

Mindfulness is a form of meditation wherein you will focus on being aware of your thoughts, feelings, and senses in the present moment without making any judgments or interpretations. There are different ways to become a more mindful person, one of which is through mindful eating. In fact, being more mindful while eating is an important aspect of intuitive eating and intuitive fasting. When you become more mindful, you will also become more aware of your surroundings and yourself.

Eating mindfully means that you are completely in the moment while doing so. Instead of simply shoveling food into your mouth, you will savor each bite of your food and each sip of your drink. Then you will chew each bite carefully while experiencing its tastes and textures. As you swallow, try to observe the food traveling down to your throat and into your stomach. This awareness will make it easier for you to observe the signals that your body is feeling about fullness and satisfaction.

In this chapter, we will focus on the mindfulness aspect of intuitive fasting along with the psychological benefits this program has to offer. Here, you will also learn how to enhance these benefits to create positive effects that last longer. You will discover the following sections:

- Mindful Eating: How This Can Help You to Eat Intuitively

- How to Eat Mindfully

- Other Ways to Listen To Your Body

If you want to follow intuitive fasting, then learning how to listen to your body is the key. This is the part you must master if you want to find success, and mindfulness can help you do this. Eating mindfully makes you more aware of the food you eat, as well as the way your body feels while you are eating. Mindfulness also helps you become more accepting of yourself and your body, which can then make you feel more positive about following the program.

Mindful Eating: How This Can Help You to Eat Intuitively

Mindful eating allows you to be present in the moment while you are eating. By practicing mindful eating, you will learn how to pay close attention to your feelings and sensations as you eat. You can taste the flavors of the food and feel the textures while you chew. You will also be able to notice your body's natural signals that indicate hunger and fullness. In addition, you will be able to observe how different types of foods affect your mood and your energy levels. You can determine which foods make you feel most satisfied and which foods often leave you wanting more. In other words, mindful eating allows you to savor your food and experience your meals in a whole new way. If you are able to do this, you will also discover that eating can become a more enjoyable experience rather than just an automatic process. Here are the other benefits of eating mindfully:

Since you will stop eating when you feel full, your digestive system won't have to work overtime to digest excess amounts of food. Therefore, mindful eating promotes better digestion.

- Even though you won't eat as much as you normally would, you will still feel full for longer periods of time because each meal will make you feel happy and satisfied. This is one of the most significant benefits that will help you break any unhealthy eating habits you may have.

- It allows you to examine your relationship with food and make changes for the better.

- It gives you some time to take a break from the stress and business of your day along with all of the negative feelings and thoughts you're having.

Mindfulness also allows you to establish a healthier connection with food, in turn allowing you to eat in a more balanced and healthier way. The best part is, you can easily incorporate mindful eating into intuitive eating. Although these two eating approaches aren't mutually exclusive, they have overlapping principles. But this doesn't mean that practicing mindfulness will already teach you to eat intuitively—you have to consciously put in an effort to combine the two in order to enhance the benefits of each.

Mindful eating and intuitive eating both focus on your mental state and how it affects your food choices. Both approaches also encourage you to learn the same practices, like enjoying your meals while you eat them and trying to notice your fullness with each bite. In addition, both approaches also help you to overcome the negative feelings you may have about food, but in different ways. For mindful eating, you will learn how to focus on your food so that you can experience and savor each bite. This transforms the activity into something enjoyable and satisfying. For intuitive eating, you will learn how to let go of thoughts like food being "the enemy," while at the same time quieting your inner food police. If you can do these things, then eating your meals becomes a more positive and fun experience.

These benefits help reduce the feelings of stress that you normally feel whenever you are eating, and this is very important since eating is a basic necessity. You need to eat in order to fuel your body. And if you start enjoying your food more, you can start focusing on nourishing your body with healthier foods without having to pressure yourself into doing so.

How to Eat Mindfully

If you want to start eating mindfully, remember that you need to perform this activity with complete awareness. This will take some practice, especially since eating is more of an automatic activity for most people—you might even be used to watching TV or scrolling through your phone while you're eating. But if you start practicing mindful eating, you need to get rid of all distractions so that you can focus on your meal. Now, let's go through some steps for you to practice mindful eating.

Reflect on Your Food Issues With Mindfulness

First of all, you need to reflect on the food issues you may have. Take some time to sit down and think about any issues like:

- not being able to control your cravings, then beating yourself up whenever you give in

- not trusting yourself enough to stop eating when there is food

- having a tendency toward "yo-yo dieting," wherein you jump from one type of diet to another because you give up quickly

- always choosing to eat the same food other people are eating just because you want to please them

These are just some examples of common food issues. You may have your own unique issues, too. Once you identify your issues, you can write them down and then use them as a reminder for what you need to change while you learn how to eat mindfully.

Gradually Get Rid of Unhealthy, Addictive Foods

While you aren't required to eliminate any foods in order to eat mindfully, it's always better to nourish your body with healthy foods. If you don't eat healthy foods, you won't know how they will make you feel. The problem with unhealthy foods is that they are often addictive, and we might confuse this addiction with feelings of satisfaction. To allow yourself to explore healthier foods, you may want to get rid of addictive foods like chocolate, cookies, pizzas, cheeseburgers, ice cream, chips, cheese, cakes, soft drinks, and french fries. If you usually have these foods in your home, you may want to stop stocking up on them. Then replace these with healthier food items that you can experiment with while you are practicing intuitive eating.

Start Using Your Senses BEFORE You Eat

Mindfulness starts even before you sit down to eat. Try to practice mindfulness as you shop for ingredients, prepare and cook your meals, and even while preparing the table by placing platefuls of food on it. As you do all of these activities, awaken your senses. Notice how different foods look, feel, and smell while you prepare them. Do the same thing while you're cooking and serving—this will prepare you for the meal itself.

Pause Before You Eat

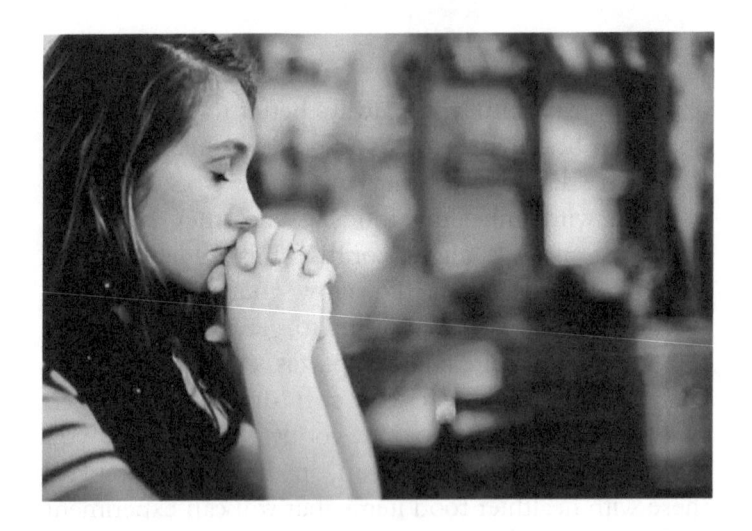

When it's finally time for you to sit down and eat, don't gobble up your food right away. Instead, take a moment to pause and prepare for your meal by calming down your body. Start by taking a couple of deep breaths. As you do this, think about the nutritional value of all the foods you have prepared. Breathing is extremely important when it comes to mindfulness. As one study revealed, breathing helps to calm your body down because there is an increase in oxygen within your body and a decrease in your heart rate (Jerath et al., 2006).

Take a Moment to Appreciate the Food in Front of You

When you feel calmer, take a moment to appreciate the food in front of you. Also, appreciate the people who prepared the meal (even if that person is you) and the people you are sharing your meal with.

Observe Yourself

Next, try to observe yourself, too. Notice your posture while sitting—you should feel relaxed while having a good posture. Notice your environment and if anything is distracting you, and try to tune those distractions out. Doing this allows you to focus on the food in front of you, which will allow you to eat more mindfully.

Tune Into Your Physical Hunger

It's important to nourish your body when you are feeling physically hungry. To do this, try to tune into your physical hunger in order to determine how hungry you are. This will help you realize if you are truly experiencing physical hunger, or if you are just giving in to strong emotions. You can consider the following to help you determine the type of hunger you are feeling:

- If you want to eat because your stomach is grumbling, you are experiencing stomach hunger.

- If you tasted a certain type of food and you want to eat more, you are experiencing mouth hunger.

- If you want to eat whenever you see food, you are experiencing eye hunger.

- If you want to eat after hearing food being cooked, you are experiencing ear hunger.

- If you want to eat when you smell food being cooked, you are experiencing nose hunger.

- If you see the time and realize that it's "time for you to eat," you are experiencing mind hunger.

- If you are experiencing strong emotions that make you want to eat, you are experiencing emotional hunger.

Tuning in to your body allows you to answer these questions accurately, which will then help you determine if you are eating for the right reasons.

Eat With Awareness

After doing all of the steps above, it's now time to start eating. As you do this, try to be mindful of each bite that you eat. Try to feel the tastes and textures of the foods as they enter your mouth. While you chew, try to notice the sensations you are feeling. While doing this, try to remain connected to your body's signals, too. This might sound odd and even challenging at first, but if you practice doing this mindfully, you will be able to awaken your own awareness.

While you are eating, you can also tune in to how the food you are eating is making you feel. If the food tastes delicious, does it make you feel happy? Does the food awaken specific emotions within you like calmness, excitement, or even anxiety? As you swallow, try to feel the food traveling down to your stomach. You can even try visualizing this. If you can do this, it will become easier for you to notice your feelings of fullness. One effective way to be more mindful while eating is by putting your utensils down between each bite.

Pause in the Middle of Your Meal

Sometime in the middle of your meal, take another pause to observe how you are feeling. This is the time to tune into your body and your hunger once again. Try to notice how the physical signs of hunger have faded away because you have already eaten a good amount of food. This is also the time to determine if you are already full, or if you need to continue eating so that you will feel full and satisfied.

Practice Mindful Reflection After Your Meal

After your meal, whether you have decided that you are full in the middle of your meal or you have finished all of the food on your plate, don't stand up right away. Take a moment to reflect on what you have eaten, how you are feeling, and if you have truly satisfied your hunger. Doing this will wrap up your mindful eating cycle nicely while leaving you with feelings of calmness and contentment.

Other Ways to Listen to Your Body

Listening to your body is an important part of mindful eating. After learning how to practice eating mindfully, the next thing to do is to find ways to listen to your body. Here are some tips to help you out.

Stop Watching Those Numbers!

If you're used to following diets, you probably focus a lot on how many calories you are consuming each day, how many pounds you have lost (or gained), how many minutes your workout routine is, and more. Living by all of these numbers can be tiring, and it also makes it difficult for you to truly listen to your body. So get rid of this habit and start focusing on the more important things!

Start Showing Respect to Your Body

In order to become more mindful, you should start treating your body with more respect and love. Think positively and start saying good things about your body. For instance, you can say things like:

- "Thank you, body, for all of the things you have done for me."

- "I trust and honor you."

- "I love my body just the way it is."

- "I respect you and I promise to care for you each day."

You can come up with your own positive affirmations to say about your body as well. This is a great way to get rid of the negativity you are feeling, while also replacing it with positive thoughts, words, and feelings.

Learn How to Awaken Your Mind-Body Connection

The easiest and most effective way to do this is through a combination of breathing and engaging your senses. After reading this, take a moment to sit down, close your eyes, and place your hand over your heart. Try to notice how your heart is beating and how your chest moves while you breathe. Now, take a deep breath, and exhale slowly. When you feel calmer, try to tune into your body. Listen to what your body is trying to tell you. Doing this regularly will make it easier for you to learn how to be more aware of your body when the need arises.

Be Aware of What Your Body Needs Right Now

Once you have tuned in to your body, ask it what you need to do to feel better. When you get your answer, make sure to honor your body's needs. For example, if your body feels thirsty, get something to drink. If your body feels hungry, get a bite to eat. If your body feels tired, get some rest. Being aware of your body's needs allows you to listen more actively so that you can satisfy your physical needs.

Find Out What Your Body Needs in the Future

It's also recommended to take some time to ask your body what it needs to heal and thrive on a long-term basis. Think about things like when you should start working out and what types of workouts you can do, if you need to change your current routine, if you need to take a day off to relax at the spa, and so on. Think of things that will improve your physical, mental, emotional, and spiritual health. Doing this will strengthen your mind-body connection, too.

Conclusion

Mindful eating doesn't have to be a challenge. In fact, it can help you learn how to calm yourself down so that you can awaken your awareness. In doing this, you will then learn how to develop your natural intuition. It's important to awaken your awareness and start listening to your body. Doing these things will connect your mind and body, which will then help you understand your own intuition.

Just like you, I had to learn and practice mindful eating. I made sure to do this regularly so that I could get used to tuning in to my body all day, every day. The more I practiced mindful eating, the more natural it felt. This will help you succeed in intuitive fasting. But as you start incorporating the other half of intuitive fasting, you need to make sure that you are always nourishing your body. One way to ensure this is by taking the right supplements. While some people use supplements to grow and develop well (like how children take vitamins), you can also use supplements to make sure that you stay healthy while you try to lose weight.

Chapter 5:

Supplements You May Wish to Consider

Vitamins and minerals are essential to your health because they help your body function optimally. Ideally, you should be getting all of these nutrients from the foods you eat—but this seldom happens. If you start fasting, though, vitamin intake becomes especially important. Following a healthy diet increases the chances of getting all of the vitamins and minerals that your body needs. As your body works to perform every individual function, both voluntary and involuntary, it needs various nutrients. These nutrients will help issue the instructions for your body to go on living.

In this chapter, you will learn about the most important supplements you need, why you need them, and how to choose the best supplements to take. It's important for you to get the right nutrients into your body so that you can keep thriving, no matter how much you change your eating patterns. Even though intuitive fasting is extremely beneficial, your body will still have to go through an adjustment period, especially at the beginning. And this adjustment period will be much easier for you with the right supplements.

Eight Supplements You Need

If you go to your local pharmacy—or even your local grocery store—to find supplements, you will see countless options. Seeing so many different types of supplements will make you feel overwhelmed. Which one do you need? Which one should you choose? Which one will help you succeed in achieving your weight loss and fitness goals?

Before we discuss the most important supplements you need, it's important to consult with your doctor first. You can even ask about the vitamins we will discuss in this chapter so that your doctor can give you a better idea of what you really need.

B-Vitamins

B-vitamins are a group of vitamins that are essential for brain function support, metabolism, the production of energy, and fatigue prevention. The B-vitamins are thiamine (B1), riboflavin (B2), niacin (B3), pantothenic acid (B5), pyridoxine (B6), biotin (B7), folic acid (B9), and cobalamin (B12). The recommended daily amount for each of these B-vitamins varies and it also varies for men and women. According to the U.S. National Institutes of Health (NIH), for men, the recommended daily amounts are:

- thiamine: 1.2 mg
- riboflavin and pyridoxine: 1.3 mg
- niacin: 16 mg
- pantothenic acid: 5 mg
- biotin: 30 micro mg
- folic acid: 400 micro mg
- cobalamin: 2.4 micro mg

For women, the recommended daily amounts are:

- thiamine and riboflavin: 1.1 mg
- niacin: 14 mg
- pantothenic acid: 5 mg
- pyridoxine: 1.3 mg
- biotin: 30 micro mg
- folic acid: 400 micro mg
- cobalamin: 2.4 micro mg

If you follow a balanced and healthy diet, you will get most of the B-vitamins you need each day. Even so, there is a possibility of developing a deficiency. When this happens, you can experience symptoms like fatigue, weakness, skin rashes, scaly skin and cracks on and around your mouth, and a swollen tongue. If left unchecked or untreated, you could experience more severe symptoms like nausea, constipation, diarrhea, tingling or numbness in your hands and feet, abdominal cramps, anemia, irritability, confusion, or even depression. B-vitamins are especially important for pregnant and breastfeeding women as they help with the growth and development of the fetus. For men, B-vitamins are also essential as they help increase testosterone levels, strength, and muscle mass.

The good news is that you can find these vitamins in many food sources such as dairy products, eggs, organ meats, red meat, chicken, fish, shellfish, dark green veggies, whole grains, beans, seeds, nuts, citrus fruits, soy products, and more. However, if you have consulted with your doctor and they recommend that you take B-vitamin supplements, make sure to take the right type of supplement. Since there are different types of B-vitamins, knowing which ones you are deficient in is key to choosing the right ones.

Magnesium

Magnesium is an essential mineral that plays an important role in more than 300 enzyme processes in the body. It helps keep the immune system safe by supporting nerve function and the regulation of blood pressure. For men, the recommended daily intake of magnesium is:

- 400 mg for those between 19 and 30 years of age
- 420 mg for those between 31 and 50 years of age
- 420 mg for those aged 51 years and above

For women, the recommended daily intake of magnesium is:

- 310 mg for those between 19 and 30 years of age
- 320 mg for those aged 31 years and above

Pregnant and breastfeeding women should increase their intake by approximately 40 mg each day throughout their pregnancy or while they are breastfeeding.

While most people don't meet these recommended daily amounts, healthy people rarely experience symptoms of magnesium deficiency. If you are deficient and you're not at the peak of your health, you may experience symptoms like appetite loss, weakness, fatigue, nausea, and vomiting. More severe symptoms may include seizures, numbness, muscle cramps, tingling sensations, spasms, changes in your heart rhythms, or even changes in your personality.

Your body needs magnesium for different things. For one, it helps you stay relaxed since magnesium helps the chemical pumps of your body work. If this doesn't happen, you will end up feeling stressed and anxious. Magnesium also stabilizes your muscles, bones, and brain. It even helps your cells produce energy, which is essential for your bodily functions.

If you want to get magnesium from the foods you eat, focus on dark leafy greens, legumes, seeds, whole grains, and nuts like cashews and almonds. You will also find this mineral in fortified foods like breakfast cereals. To find the right magnesium supplements for your needs, consult with your doctor first. It's also important to follow the recommended dosage when taking magnesium supplements so that you don't overdose on this mineral.

Multivitamins

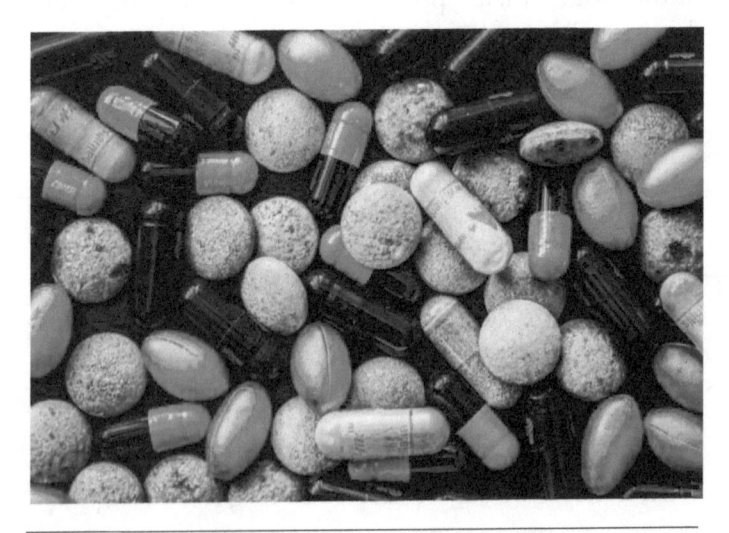

Multivitamins contain different types of vitamins and minerals along with other healthy ingredients. It's even more challenging to choose multivitamins because the contents vary from one product and brand to another—they come in different forms like powders, capsules, tablets, liquids, and even chewable gummies.

If you go through the ingredients lists of multivitamins, you will see that most of them contain the basic nutrients the body needs like B-vitamins, Vitamin C, Vitamin D, magnesium, zinc, and more. The main benefit of multivitamins is that they allow you to take different types of vitamins and minerals at the same time. This means that if you are deficient in several nutrients, you can try to find multivitamins that contain all of the nutrients you need. Once again, you should ask your doctor first before taking these supplements.

Omega-3 Supplements

Omega-3 fatty acids are essential for your overall health and well-being, which is why these supplements are considered one of the most important. Omega-3 fatty acids are a group of polyunsaturated fats that your body doesn't produce naturally. But since they are essential, you need to get your omega-3s from various dietary sources. There are three types of omega-3 fatty acids, which are: docosahexaenoic acid (DHA), alpha-linolenic acid (ALA), and eicosapentaenoic acid (EPA).

Omega-3 fatty acids offer many health benefits. For one, they are very effective at reducing inflammation, which is a major factor in the development of chronic diseases. These fatty acids can also improve heart health along with various conditions like Crohn's disease, rheumatoid arthritis, fatty liver disease, high cholesterol levels, and even cancer. It can even be helpful for those who suffer from mental conditions like ADHD, anxiety, dementia, and depression.

You can find ALA in plant-based oils like soybean, canola, and flaxseed along with nuts and seeds like walnuts and chia seeds. As for EPA and DHA, these are commonly found in fish like anchovies, sardines, salmon, and other types of seafood. When it comes to choosing omega-3 supplements, try to avoid processed products. For instance, fish oil is one of the best types of omega-3 supplements. But when choosing such a product, make sure to check the purity of the product. Also, you need to store such products well as they can easily get rancid.

Probiotics

Probiotics are a type of bacteria that help promote the health of your gut. Our bodies have good and bad bacteria. The former helps maintain gut health while the latter causes inflammation or disease. By taking probiotic supplements, you can increase the good bacteria in your body. This, in turn, can improve your overall health while helping prevent inflammatory bowel diseases (IBD), diarrhea, and irritable bowel syndrome. These good bacteria can also prevent yeast infections, urinary tract infections, eczema and other skin conditions, respiratory and stomach infections, asthma, and other types of allergies. Also, taking certain types of probiotic supplements can even improve your weight loss efforts.

When choosing probiotic supplements, check the reputation of the brand. Make sure to purchase from a trustworthy brand, preferably one that has performed third-party testing on its products. Also, high-quality probiotic supplements should at least contain B. breve, B. bifidum, B. longum, L. acidophilus, L. casei, L. reuteri, L. rhamnosus, and S. thermophilus. These are the probiotic strains that are commonly found in healthy people.

Vitamin C

Vitamin C is a type of antioxidant that helps your body fight disease and prevent cell damage. This is the most common vitamin supplement you will find. It's also one of the most effective and safest nutrients out there. This vitamin has tons of benefits. It helps reduce your blood pressure and cholesterol levels. It also helps your body absorb iron more effectively and helps your blood carry oxygen, too. This antioxidant is especially beneficial to the immune system, which then makes sure that your body is strong enough to combat injuries, infections, and illnesses.

You can get Vitamin C from citrus fruits and different kinds of vegetables like carrots, broccoli, kale, and spinach. Since Vitamin C is quite common in the healthiest foods you should be eating (fruits and veggies), you can get all of the Vitamin C you need from your diet. But if you do need Vitamin C supplements, you can find these easily because they are the most common. Opt for supplements that come from trusted brands. You can get supplements that only contain Vitamin C, or multivitamins that contain this essential vitamin, too.

Vitamin D

Vitamin D is a type of fat-soluble vitamin that your body produces naturally. When you expose yourself to sunlight, your body produces even more of this vitamin. Vitamin D has many important functions, the most significant of which is the regulation of phosphorus and calcium absorption in the body. This is essential for the optimal function of your immune system.

Since Vitamin D is produced by your body, you don't have to rely on dietary sources as much. Just make sure that you get enough sunlight so that your body continues to produce this vitamin. Generally, you need between 15 to 20 micro mg of Vitamin D to ensure your health and your body's optimal functioning. If your body doesn't produce Vitamin D, you will be at risk for chronic inflammation. In more severe cases, you might also end up suffering from calcium deficiency. Other symptoms include a compromised immune system, weakness, aches, pains, fatigue, and even stress fractures. You would have to get a blood test to determine if you are deficient in Vitamin D. In such a case, you can start taking Vitamin D supplements at the advice of your doctor. You can also increase your intake of Vitamin D-rich foods like fortified milk, sardines, salmon, beef liver, shrimp, yogurt, and eggs (specifically the yolks).

Zinc Supplements

Zinc is a mineral that your body needs to combat viruses and bacteria. It's also responsible for the production of genetic material (DNA), and it helps ensure that your body works the way it should. Men need around 11 mg of zinc each day while women need around 8 mg. For women who are pregnant or breastfeeding, they need to increase their intake to 12 mg.

This mineral is essential, as being deficient in zinc can increase your risk of infertility and diabetes. It can also cause symptoms like appetite loss, hair loss, sores on the skin and eyes, and even diarrhea. When it comes to getting your zinc from dietary sources, the best options include oysters, lean red meat, Alaskan king crab, chicken (especially dark meat), and cashews. Before taking a zinc supplement, consult with your doctor first. There are many types of zinc supplements available, and your doctor can help you choose the best one to improve your health.

Conclusion

Supplements are very important since they can help you make sure that you are getting the right nutrition. As I started my intuitive fasting journey, I did notice that my body was undergoing some changes. To make sure that I was putting myself first, I consulted with my doctor. Although I wanted to lose weight and become healthier in the long run, I didn't want to put myself in a situation where I wasn't nourishing my body properly—I knew that this would have adverse consequences.

My doctor talked to me about taking some supplements. This is when I started researching the most essential supplements and how to find the right ones. Now that you have an idea of what supplements you can take to ensure your health, you can now focus on starting your own intuitive fasting journey. And this is what you will learn in the next chapters.

Chapter 6:

Phase 1: Starting Intuitive Fasting

Fasting is a process where you deprive your body of food for a specific amount of time and for a specific purpose. For instance, fasting for religious purposes is very common. But it's also commonly done by people who want to lose weight. Since you're interested in intuitive fasting, then you may also want to lose weight. Of course, this isn't the only benefit you can gain from intuitive fasting.

After learning all about the two core diets that intuitive fasting consists of, it's now time to learn how to start your own intuitive fasting program. In this chapter, you will learn what to do in the first week of intuitive fasting. You will discover the following sections:

- What is the 12:12 Fast?
- Making Healthy Food Choices
- Sample Daily Routine

- Incorporating Intuitive Eating

- Does it Really Work?

As you go through the information here, you might feel a bit overwhelmed. But as someone who has tried this program and succeeded, I can tell you that it's a lot easier than it looks. So keep that positive mindset and let's continue!

What is the 12:12 Fast?

The 12:12 fast is one of the many IF methods that you can follow. This method is ideal for beginners, since it allows you to eat for 12 hours and fast for the other 12 hours. In other words, each day you will only be eating for half a day. Following this method every day will force your body into ketosis. This is when your body starts converting fat (even stored fat) into energy while releasing ketones into your bloodstream. When this happens, your body transforms into a fat-burning machine, which is why weight loss is one of the most common benefits.

When you follow this method, you can choose how many meals you will eat in your 12-hour eating window. Just make sure that you finish your last meal of the day before your 12 hours are up. If this is your first time fasting, you will experience hunger pains once your fasting window starts (or sometime in the middle of your fasting window). This is normal. If you stick with the program, your body will adjust to fasting over time. If you don't think you can last for 12 hours without eating anything, you can even add an extra week to the program. Start a week earlier and try to fast for about 10 hours a day. This will help you transition into the 12:12 method easily. The important thing is to get used to not eating for long periods of time. But you shouldn't force yourself to endure your hunger pains, as this might make the experience a negative one.

Another way to make the 12:12 fast easier is by scheduling your fasting time wisely. To make your fasting windows more bearable, schedule them at the same time when you sleep. For instance, if you have a 9-to-5 day job, you can schedule your fasting period at night. If you sleep for 8 hours each night, that means you would only have to endure 4 more hours of fasting! But if you work at night and sleep during the day, then you can schedule your fasting window in the morning and have your eating window at night. This is a very strategic and practical way to find success with the 12:12 fast.

As part of the intuitive fasting program, you will be doing the 12:12 fast for one whole week. It's important to create a routine and stick with it, as this will prepare you for the next weeks of the program. It's also important to remember that you are following an intuitive fasting program, not IF. This means that you should also start incorporating the principles of mindful eating and intuitive eating while you are getting used to your new routine.

This is what makes intuitive fasting more effective compared to other weight loss diets. Instead of just focusing on the timing of your meals, you will also focus on learning how to listen to your body and eat more mindfully.

Making Healthy Food Choices

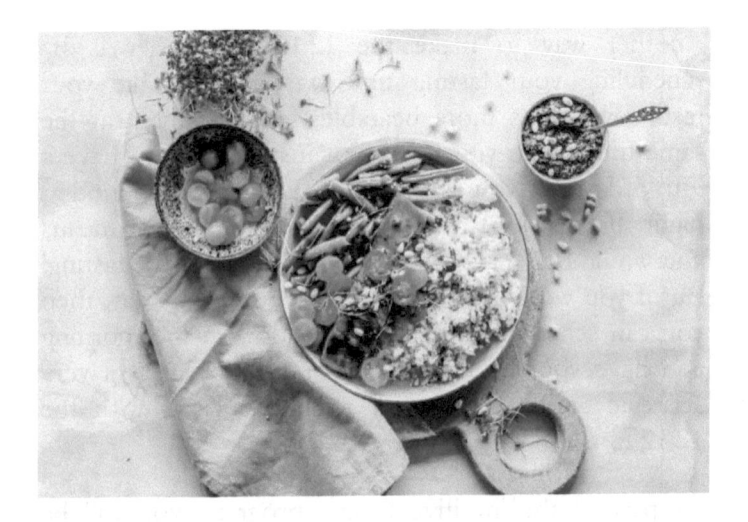

When you start your intuitive fasting program, try not to think of it as depriving yourself. Instead, think of your new eating approach as a way for you to lose weight and become healthier. To make this process easier and ensure that you will get all the benefits of the program, try to consume nutritious and satisfying foods throughout your eating window. This includes lean proteins, complex carbohydrates, and healthy fats. If you can, try to avoid refined sugar and refined carbs as these will just mess up your sugar levels. To give you an idea of the best foods to include in your diet, here are some examples:

- Avocados are highly recommended, because they contain healthy fats and are very filling. This fruit is also very versatile since you can add it to sweet and savory dishes.

- Berries are nature's candy and they are rich in Vitamin C. If you're craving something sweet, you should snack on a handful of berries. You can also use these healthy treats in different types of desserts, too.

- Eggs contain protein and healthy fats, both of which are essential to your health. Eating eggs will keep you satisfied for long periods of time.

- Fermented foods like sauerkraut, kefir, and kombucha are rich in probiotics. Eating these once in a while will also be beneficial to your health.

- Fish (especially fatty fish) are rich in protein, Vitamin D, and omega-3s. There are many types of fish to choose from and you can cook them in different ways.

- Legumes and beans contain high-fiber, low-calorie carbs making them another amazing addition to your meals. You can also add these foods to various dishes to make them healthier and more filling.

- Nuts and seeds are also great options because they contain healthy fats. You can snack on these on their own or add them to sweet and savory dishes.

- Vegetables definitely belong to your diet. There are so many types out there, and they will make your meals more interesting. Aside from leafy greens, you can also opt for more filling veggies like Brussels sprouts, cauliflower, and broccoli. Potatoes are another versatile vegetable that you can add to your diet. But instead of indulging in potato chips and fries, opt for healthier options like mashed, roasted, or boiled potatoes.

- Whole grains contain protein and fiber, which will make you feel full. These foods will also increase your metabolic rate, which can help enhance your weight loss efforts.

These are just some examples of the healthiest options to add to your meals. By incorporating these foods, your meals will become more satisfying, which means that fasting won't be as difficult. When it's time for you to fast, you can stay hydrated by drinking lots of water and some calorie-free drinks like plain coffee or tea. If you want a more refreshing beverage, you can add some cucumber or lemon slices—or even mint leaves—to your glass of water. Remember that intuitive fasting is all about flexibility. You can create your own unique meal plan that will make you happy and satisfied.

Sample Daily Routine

No matter what type of fasting method you will start with, the best way to increase your success is by starting gradually. Even for intuitive fasting, you don't have to begin with the 12:12 fast right away. You can add 1 to 2 weeks prior to your program to help your body get used to fasting. For instance, you can start by fasting for 10 hours for a week, then move it up to 11 hours for another week. When you start your first week of the program, you can transition into fasting for 12 hours a day.

Doing this will give your body and mind time to adjust to your new routine. And if you can time your fasting and eating windows strategically, that would be even better. For example, if you always eat a hearty breakfast every morning, you can start to practice fasting by delaying your usual breakfast time by about 30 minutes. The next day, delay it by an hour. Keep doing this until you reach the timing you want for your 12-hour fasting window. Another way to increase your chances of success on the 12:12 fast is by sticking to a routine. After you have trained your body to get used to fasting, choose a schedule. For example, you can set your eating window from 8:00 a.m. to 8:00 p.m. Based on this schedule, you can come up with a plan such as this one:

- At 8:00 a.m., break your fast with a bowl of oatmeal or a healthy, homemade smoothie to start your day.

- At 9:00 a.m., take a stroll outside for about half an hour. Remember that exposure to sunlight can help your body produce Vitamin D.

- If you're feeling hungry, you can have a light snack like a handful of nuts or a small bowl of fresh berries.

- When 12:00 noon comes along, you can enjoy a nutritious and filling lunch like a root veggie salad with a side of couscous.

- At 3:00 p.m., you can enjoy another healthy snack like dark chocolate, peanut butter, or an apple.

- And at 7:00 p.m., enjoy your last meal of the day—something filling and healthy like beef stew with veggies and potatoes.

At 8:00 p.m., you should already be done with all of your meals. This is when your fasting window starts. Remember to drink a lot of water and stick with other non-caloric drinks. When it's time for you to sleep, you can relax and allow your body to repair itself while you rest.

Again, this is just an example of what a typical day would look like if you are following the 12:12 fast. You don't have to stick with strict timings, especially since you will be incorporating intuitive eating into your program. This means that you have to listen to your body's physical hunger signals so that you can nourish your body whenever you are hungry, not just because you feel bored or anxious about the eating program you have just started.

Incorporating Intuitive Eating

As you follow the first week of the intuitive eating program, you shouldn't just focus on the timing aspect. Remember that the 12-hour fasting and 12-hour eating windows are just one part of intuitive fasting. You also have to start practicing the intuitive eating part as well. Let's go through the core principles of intuitive eating once again along with some tips for how to incorporate these principles into your new routine:

- **Get Rid of the Diet Mentality**

As you begin your program, don't think of it as "another one of those diets" that you have tried and failed at. This is a program that will teach you how to listen to your body, nourish yourself in the best possible ways, and change the way your body works through fasting.

- **Honor the Hunger You Feel**

When you are allowed to eat, never starve yourself. This means that when you feel physical hunger at any point during your eating window, eat something. You can manage your cravings by eating smaller meals throughout the day. It's also a good idea to keep healthy snacks at home so that you don't resort to unhealthy, yet convenient, options.

- **Stop Seeing Food as the Enemy**

In the same way, you shouldn't consider food as "the enemy," whether on your fasting or eating windows. During your eating windows, use food to nourish your body. During your fasting periods, try not to think about food all the time. Instead, find fun things to distract yourself.

- **Challenge Your Inner Food Police**

During your eating windows, your inner food police should take a break. You don't have to feel guilty about eating, especially since this is the time when you're allowed to eat. But when your fasting window comes along, your food police can go "on duty"—only to remind you that it's time to fast, though, so you should only focus on keeping yourself hydrated.

- **Recognize and Respect Your Feelings of Fullness**

Even during your eating windows, you don't have to eat excessively. Go back to mindful eating so that you can listen to your body while you eat. When you feel full, stop eating. Don't worry about the time. You can always eat again when you feel hungry, as long as you're still in your eating window.

- **Discover What Makes You Feel Satisfied**

This is one of the most enjoyable parts of the process. Try different foods out to discover what makes you feel happy and satisfied. If you feel this way after eating, then your fasting windows won't be too difficult. Make your diet interesting by trying different foods and observing how each food makes you feel, both physically and emotionally.

- **Accept Your Feelings and Cope Without Using Food**

As you learn your body's physical hunger signals, you will also be able to determine when you are feeling emotional hunger. In such a case, accept your feelings, then try to find an activity to help you cope with those feelings.

- **Accept, Respect, and Love Your Body**

As you go through each day of your intuitive fasting program, you will rely on your body to keep going, even during your fasting windows. Keep yourself inspired and motivated by learning to accept, respect, and love your body. This will make the whole program a positive experience for you, which will then make things much easier and more enjoyable.

- **Get Moving and Feel the Difference**

In the sample daily routine in the previous section, you may have noticed that there is a part where you take a short walk outside. To enhance your weight loss efforts and make your intuitive fasting program more effective, try incorporating physical activity into your routine. You don't have to start an intense workout. Things like taking strolls, walking up and down staircases, or even cleaning your house can already count as physical activities. By moving around, you will definitely feel the difference in a good way!

- **Focus On Gentle Nutrition**

By nourishing your body with healthy, nutrient-dense foods, you will increase your chances of succeeding in this program. The reason for this is that healthy foods will provide your body with the nutrients it needs to stay strong, healthy, and able. Although you don't have to force yourself to eat certain foods or restrict yourself from eating foods that you used to love, changing your diet gradually by making healthier food choices will already go a long way toward helping you lose weight.

Keep these things in mind as you follow the first week of your intuitive fasting program. Then continue to incorporate these principles as you enter your second, third, and fourth weeks to make sure that you're following the program well.

Does it Really Work?

Yes, it does.

As you now know, I have followed this program from start to finish and it helped me lose weight. The best part about this program is that by the end of it, I had learned how to eat healthily. I never felt pressured, and I never felt like I had to restrict myself at any point throughout my journey. But I am not the only one who has found success. Many of my friends and clients have also found success by following intuitive fasting. I have even read tons of success stories online and some of them have really stood out.

One such story is from a fitness editor who often writes about different types of diets. She aims to educate people on how they can reach their health goals, but she hadn't really followed a specific diet until she learned about the 12:12 fasting method. She tried it out and found it to be extremely effective. Through this eating method, she discovered some important things about herself:

- At the beginning of the diet, she felt very hungry. She jumped right into the diet and it took a toll on her body, especially since she was also working. But after 10 days, those feelings of extreme hunger started going away. That's when things started to get easier. This is why it's important to start gradually, especially if you're new at fasting.

- She also discovered that she had bloating issues, especially after eating lots of grains and dairy. Since she became more conscious of what she was eating, she was able to discover something new about her body. This knowledge allowed her to get rid of her bloating issues by making sure to only eat grains and dairy in moderation.

- Finally, she also realized that she had broken her habit of mindlessly snacking. By following a 12-hour eating routine, she made sure that her meals always counted, which then helped her avoid snacking even though she wasn't hungry.

Discovering new things about yourself and your body is another thing that I love about intuitive fasting. During this first week, you will realize that fasting doesn't have to be a difficult thing. Instead, it will be one of the best changes you will make in your life that will help you lose weight while improving your overall health.

Conclusion

The first week of your intuitive fasting program will go by quickly, especially as you try to incorporate the best aspects of intermittent fasting and intuitive eating. With each day, your body will get used to not eating for 12 hours. In the process, you will also start familiarizing yourself with your body's natural hunger signals. If you have finished this week, congratulate yourself on it! Then you can gear up for the second week of your program, where you will increase your fasting window and find new ways to deal with your feelings of hunger. Keep going!

Chapter 7:

Phase 2: Getting the Hang of It

After you have followed the 12:12 fasting method for one whole week, it's time to move on to your second week. This is where things will get a little bit challenging, as you will increase your fasting window to 16 hours. Since your eating window will be significantly shorter, you have to be even more observant of your hunger signals. In the first 1 or 2 days, you will still be used to having 12 hours to satisfy your hunger. But now, you will have 4 hours less. So you really need to tune into your body so that you won't end up feeling extremely hungry once your fasting window begins. The 16:8 IF method is endorsed by celebrities, influencers, and even health experts because of all the benefits you can gain from it. These include:

- It reduces the effects of oxidative stress on your body.

- It gives your body a break by benefiting your vital organs, metabolic functions, digestive system, and absorptive hormones.

- It decreases inflammation in your body, which then lowers your risk of developing chronic diseases.

In this chapter, you will discover what you need to do for the second week of your intuitive fasting program. Here, we will focus on the 16:8 method and how you can stay on track throughout the week. The sections included that we will discuss here are:

- What is the 16:8 Fasting Method?

- What are Its Benefits?

- Healthy Food Choices

- Tips to Help Fight Hunger Pains

During my second week, I felt more confident about my ability to follow a routine. The first week allowed me to get a feel of what fasting is all about and how to fix my routine to make the process as easy as possible. You can do this too! Although the longer fasting period might seem overwhelming, if you plan for it and you know how to fight those stubborn hunger pains, you will be able to succeed and move forward.

What Is the 16:8 Fasting Method?

The 16:8 method of fasting involves cycling between 8 hours of eating and 16 hours of fasting. This means that in the second week of your intuitive fasting program, you will only eat for 8 hours each day, then only drink water and non-caloric beverages for the other 16 hours. If you are following IF, you can do this method as often as you want each week. But since you are following the intuitive fasting program, you will be following this method for one whole week.

This method of fasting is one of the most popular for those following IF. Although it's not ideal for beginners, those who have succeeded in the less intense methods often take their IF journey further by following the 16:8 method. This method has also grown in popularity because it is very effective in helping people burn fat and lose weight. If you were able to stick with the first week of your intuitive fasting program, then transitioning into this method will be easier compared to if you start with the 16:8 method right away. Just like with the 12:12 fast, you need to choose a time window for this method. Since your eating window here will be 8 hours long, you can choose what time to start so that you can count the hours and determine what time this window will end. Some of the most popular time windows for this method are:

- 7: 00 a.m. to 3:00 p.m.

- 9:00 a.m. to 5:00 p.m.

- 12:00 noon to 8:00 p.m.

- 2:00 p.m. to 10:00 p.m.

Of course, these are just suggestions. You can come up with your own schedule depending on your daily routine. You can even base your eating window on the schedule you followed during your first week. For instance, if your 12:12 fasting schedule was 8:00 a.m. to 8:00 p.m., you can simply adjust your starting or ending time. This would give you an eating window of:

- 8:00 a.m. to 4:00 p.m.

- 9:00 a.m. to 5:00 p.m.

- 10:00 a.m. to 6:00 p.m.

The great thing about following this method is its flexibility. You can choose your own timing so that you don't have to feel like you are following a strict schedule that is imposed on you. Make sure the schedule you choose fits your lifestyle and your daily routine. That way, you don't have to make any drastic changes to your work or home life just to accommodate your new eating program.

During your daily eating window, make sure to nourish yourself with the right foods. Even if you are in your second week, you should still remember the principles of intuitive eating. Continue to listen to your body and awaken your awareness at every meal. You can also continue experimenting with different types of foods, then keep making notes about your observations. If you lead a very busy life, you can even set a timer for the start and end of your eating window so that you can start on time and have your last meal before your eating window ends.

What Are Its Benefits?

Just like the 12:12 fast, the 16:8 method is very simple. As long as you have set your schedule, you can simply follow it throughout the week. During your eating window, you can enjoy 1 to 3 meals (or even several small meals) throughout. But if you plan your meals carefully and you can cook nutrient-dense meals that contain all of the food groups that comprise a healthy diet, then you can just have 1 to 2 full, satisfying meals during your eating window without worrying about not getting the recommended daily amounts of nutrients your body needs. Shifting to the 16:8 method in your second week offers more health benefits including:

- Your body will become more efficient at fat-burning since your fasting time will be longer. Since ketosis only happens when you are fasting, you will be able to burn more fat each day compared to the previous week.

- Since your body will become more powerful at burning fat, you may also lose more weight. This is especially true if you stick with the program and try to focus on nourishing your body with the right foods.

- The 'break' your body gets through fasting helps balance your hormone levels, which then optimizes their functions.

- There is an increase in the stimulation of your stem cells, an improvement in your cholesterol levels, and a stabilization in your blood sugar levels.

- Your overall body composition improves, which then lowers your risk of heart disease, chronic illnesses, and even cancer.

You can even end up looking more youthful as all of these benefits can help delay the process of aging! Try to keep these benefits in mind to keep you motivated throughout your second week when you will follow the 16:8 method.

Before I started following intuitive fasting, I also felt unhappy with my health. I wanted to lose weight and become healthier. When I learned about this program, I realized that it was offering everything I needed. And when I started following it, I discovered that—unlike other diets—this one actually delivered. With each week, I noticed good changes happening to me. I had to put in the effort to increase my awareness while following the diet; but the more I practiced, the easier it became. As I approached the last few days of my second week, I was ready and motivated to continue with the next week of the program... and you can do it, too!

Healthy Food Choices

If you want to make the most of the health benefits mentioned above, you should focus on nourishing your body with healthy, nutrient-dense foods. While you don't have to eliminate entire food groups from your diet just so you can lose weight, remember that you only have 8 hours to feed your body. If you only eat unhealthy foods throughout those 8 hours and you do this every day for a week, you might end up feeling some adverse side effects instead of improvements to your health.

Since you have a limited time to eat, encourage yourself to focus on whole foods that will make you feel full and satisfied. When you fill-up on nutrient-rich foods, you won't feel as hungry during your fasting window as compared to filling up on junk foods that contain empty calories. When planning your meals for this second week of your intuitive eating program, focus on foods like:

- **Fruits**

Fruits are nature's candy. Aside from helping you satisfy your sweet tooth, fruits contain plenty of essential nutrients that your body needs to stay healthy. There are so many types of fruits out there like apples, berries, bananas, citrus fruits, pears, peaches, grapes, avocados, and more.

- **Healthy Fats**

Get rid of the notion that fats are "the enemy," because your body needs fats to stay healthy. The key here is to choose food sources that contain healthy fats like avocados, fatty fish, and olive oil.

- **Proteins**

Protein sources should be included in your diet, too, since these are filling and they will help prevent muscle loss while you are fasting. Just try not to eat too much protein, as this can be broken down by your body and converted into glucose. When this happens, your body cannot achieve ketosis wherein it starts burning fat. Also, opt for healthy protein sources like legumes, eggs, lean meat, nuts, seeds, poultry, and more.

- **Vegetables**

While you are following the intuitive fasting program, eating lots of vegetables is essential. These nutritional powerhouses will provide you with essential nutrients; and they also contain fiber, which can help you feel full for longer periods of time. Some great examples of veggies include leafy greens, cruciferous vegetables, root vegetables, and more.

- **Whole Grains**

Just like vegetables, whole grains will make your meals more filling, giving them a much-needed nutrient boost. Opt for grains like quinoa, barley, oats, and buckwheat as these are very versatile and satisfying.

These are some examples of the best foods to include in your diet. It's also recommended to avoid foods that are ultra-processed such as frozen meals, deep-fried foods, packaged snacks, and sugary drinks. Of course, these are just suggestions for you to maximize the effects of your eating program. As always, you should keep yourself hydrated during your fasting window by drinking a lot of water and other non-caloric beverages.

When you are planning your meals while following intuitive fasting, remember to trust your intuition. Think about what types of foods will make you feel satisfied, even if you enter your daily fasting window. You don't have to count your calories and you don't have to restrict yourself from eating certain foods. Stick with good-sized portions—and while you eat, always remember to look out for your natural feelings of fullness.

Tips to Help Fight Hunger Pains

Focusing on healthful eating while following the 16:8 method is key to a smooth transition, while it also increases your chances of experiencing the different benefits. Plus, if you only eat unhealthy foods like junk food or fast food, these could actually contribute to weight gain while increasing your risk of developing various diseases. These are the opposite effects of what you want. So it's best to focus on your nutrition while still allowing yourself to indulge in your cravings once in a while.

As you follow the 16:8 method in your second week, one of the biggest challenges you will encounter is hunger. Even though your body has already adjusted to not eating anything for 12 hours a day, you will still add 4 hours to your fasting window during this second week. Although drinking water and other non-caloric beverages can help alleviate your hunger, you might feel hunger more often than before. To make this second week much easier for you, here are some tips to fight those inevitable hunger pains:

- **Drink Water Throughout the Day**

Water is the most important beverage to drink while following intuitive fasting. You need water to keep yourself hydrated, and you also need water to give you a feeling of fullness—especially during your fasting periods. It's best to drink water at regular intervals throughout the day rather than drinking large amounts of water only during your fasting window. Make it a habit to drink water regularly so that you won't be in danger of getting dehydrated at any point during the day.

- **Try Cinnamon Herbal Tea**

Cinnamon herbal tea is a non-caloric beverage that you can drink during your fasting window. It's actually recommended to drink this tea, as it can help suppress your appetite. Whenever you feel hungry, brew a cup of this tea for yourself and enjoy it while reading a book or spending some time outside.

- **Exercise Right Before or Sometime in the Middle of Your Eating Window**

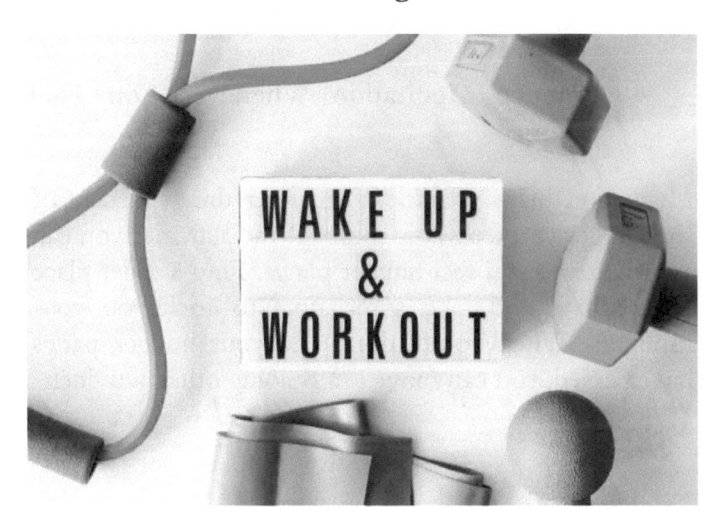

The great thing about exercise is that it can help you lose weight and it can also trigger your hunger. This is important, since you will be listening to your body's natural hunger signals. You can exercise an hour before your eating window starts so that you will feel hungry at the right time. Or, you can exercise somewhere in the middle of your eating window so you will feel hungry right before your fasting window begins.

- **Reduce the Time You Spend in Front of the TV**

While watching TV can potentially distract you from the hunger you feel, it can also cause you distress. We often see many images of food on TV from commercials, TV shows, movies, and more. The more you see these images of mouthwatering meals, the hungrier you will feel! Try to find other things to do that will make you feel relaxed and happy.

- **Practice Meditation Whenever You Feel Hungry**

Meditation helps you focus on other things instead of the hunger you feel. This is one of the activities you can do whenever you feel hunger pangs. Find a quiet place to meditate and take some time to focus on your thoughts. When you're done and your hunger pangs have passed, you can move on to doing other activities.

- **Remember to Eat Mindfully During Your Eating Window**

Eating mindfully makes your meals more relaxing and enjoyable. Since you only have a few hours to eat your meals, this is key to helping you feel more satisfied after every meal. Whether you are eating a snack or a full meal, eating mindfully during your eating windows will make it easier to endure your fasting windows.

As you can see, there are many ways to deal with hunger during your fasting window. But you should still tune in to your body so that you can recognize your feelings of hunger. This way, you can determine if you truly are physically hungry or the changes you are making to your eating patterns are awakening your emotional hunger.

Conclusion

The second week of your intuitive eating program may seem overwhelming, but with everything you have learned in this chapter, you should know that it's totally doable. As always, try to stay positive throughout the process. Do this by focusing on learning how to listen to your body while planning the meals you will eat during the hours you are allowed to eat. At this point, you should already have a better idea of how intermittent fasting and intuitive eating work together. Since you can adjust the timing to your own schedule, this makes the eating program much easier and more sustainable. You're already halfway there! Now it is time to move on to the next week of your journey, where you will push your body further in order to achieve the results you are looking for.

Chapter 8:

Phase 3: Pushing Toward Success

After two weeks of following the intuitive fasting program, your body should have already adjusted to fasting. If you have been following a routine for the past weeks, good for you. And if you were able to stick with the fasting methods, you should congratulate yourself!

As your second week of intuitive fasting comes to an end, it's time to start thinking about the next week, which is where you will challenge yourself even more. When you start your third week of the intuitive fasting program, you will follow the One Meal a Day plan, or OMAD. As the name implies, this means that you will only eat one meal once a day for seven days. To find out how to do this, you will learn the following in the sections ahead:

- What is OMAD?
- What Can I Eat?

- The Benefits of OMAD

- Are There Any Risks?

When I began my intuitive fasting program, I already knew that I would have to follow the OMAD diet. Of course, I felt quite intimidated at first. But after two weeks of following my fasting routine, I knew that I would be able to follow this diet, too. I was more confident about my ability to nourish my body with healthy foods and endure my hunger throughout my daily fasting windows. I also prepared by finding different ways to ease my hunger pangs, which then made this week a lot easier for me. And you can do this, too.

What Is OMAD?

The One Meal a Day diet is more commonly known as the OMAD diet. This involves only eating one meal each day. It also means that the diet involves significant caloric restriction, which is why weight loss is one of the main benefits of this diet. Since you will only eat one meal each day, your body will be forced into ketosis after it has broken down what you've eaten. Since you will not be eating anything else throughout the day, your body will then resort to burning your fat stores. This is considered the most intense IF method, but it also involves cycling between periods of eating and periods of fasting.

Depending on how long it takes you to eat your single meal for the day, your fasting window would be somewhere between 22 to 23 hours. Just like all the other IF methods, OMAD changes the way your body breaks down and uses nutrients for fuel. When you follow a "normal diet," wherein you eat three meals a day plus one or two snacks, your body will get its energy from the food that you eat throughout the day. In particular, your body breaks down the carbohydrates you eat and converts them into glucose. Unfortunately, if you consume too much food or you eat too often throughout the day, you will end up having more glucose in your body than what you need. When this happens, the insulin in your body will carry the extra glucose to your fat cells for storage.

Through fasting, your body will produce less insulin. Since your body still needs energy to fuel all of your bodily functions, your fat cells will start releasing energy to keep things moving. But this will only happen if you fast long enough for your insulin levels to decrease. Of course, if you follow OMAD, you will definitely reach that point wherein your body will start burning fat for fuel.

As with all other IF methods, OMAD doesn't restrict how much food or what types of food you should eat. But if you want to follow this diet safely and gain all of its benefits, you need to make sure that you nourish your body with all of the nutrients it needs through that one meal. It's also recommended to eat your meal at the same time each day. This ensures that you will have a consistent fasting period for the whole week. After following OMAD for a few days, you will notice that you will feel hunger at the same time each day. This is more likely to happen if you have a routine. It's also important to stay hydrated all day, every day.

Realistically speaking, it's not possible to consume all of the calories you need in a single meal. In general, the recommended daily caloric intake is 2,000 calories for women and 2,500 calories for men. Do you think you can eat that much in a single meal? Even if you can, this isn't recommended. Instead, you should make sure that each calorie in your meal counts. You can do this by eating healthy, nutrient-dense foods.

What Can I Eat?

The OMAD diet is quite intense, so you should focus more on your nutrition during this week. Although you can technically eat anything you want, you can get the most out of this diet if you make healthy food choices. For instance, having a tray of fast food for your meal is fine, but you would feel more satisfied if you prepare a salad for yourself that's loaded with whole grains, beans, roasted vegetables, seeds, nuts, and some feta cheese—with a roasted salmon filet on the side. Not only will you feel better about your meal, but you will also feel more satisfied after eating such a dish.

Since you will only be eating one meal a day, you will consume fewer calories for the whole week than you usually would. This feature of the OMAD diet will help you lose weight. Following this diet isn't as easy as following the 12:12 and 16:8 methods, though. But if you are able to awaken your intuitiveness and mindfulness, you can help yourself get through the week without falling off the wagon or binging on all the unhealthy foods in your home. Again, the key here is to plan your meals well so that you will feel full for a longer period of time. Here are some of the best food options to include in your diet:

- **Avocados**

Avocados are nutritious, versatile, and super satisfying. You can add avocados to salads and other types of dishes for a nutrient boost and the addition of a wonderful savory texture.

- **Berries**

Adding something sweet to your meal will make it even more satisfying, while also making you feel happier, too. You can whip up a dessert with berries or simply add a handful of berries to your meal. Either way, these nutritious fruits are a valuable addition to your diet.

- **Dark Chocolate**

This is another tasty option to have at the end of your meal. Dark chocolate is high in healthy fats and fiber, which makes it quite healthy as well. Just try not to go overboard when it comes to eating this indulgent treat!

- **Eggs**

Eggs are high in protein and they can be cooked in different ways. Cook your eggs a different way each day, then add them to your meal to leave you feeling full and satisfied.

- **Legumes**

There are many types of legumes to choose from such as lentils, chickpeas, and beans. All of these are high in fiber, which means that your body will take a longer time to digest them. Add legumes to stews, soups, and salads to accompany your main meal.

- **Nuts and Seeds**

This is another food group that offers so many choices. Aside from adding nuts to various dishes, you can also add a handful of nuts to your meal for the day. Nuts are rich in healthy fats and other nutrients to help you feel full after eating.

- **Salmon**

This is one of the healthiest fish on the planet, and it definitely belongs in your diet. Although you don't have to eat salmon every day, adding this fish to your meal as the main source of protein is recommended as it is also high in omega-3s.

- **Whole Grains**

This is another excellent addition to your one meal for the day. There are different types of whole grains to choose from, and adding them to your meals will make them more filling and nutrient-dense. Try to focus on unprocessed whole grains, as these are much healthier and more satisfying.

Apart from these examples, you can also add any other foods to your meal for the day. Adding different kinds of foods to your plate will help ensure that you are still getting all of the nutrients you need each day, even if you are only eating a single meal. Also, remember to keep yourself hydrated throughout your fasting window just as you did with the first two weeks of your program.

It's only natural to feel hungrier during this week, since your fasting window will be significantly longer. Just continue to listen to your body so that you can determine what you want to eat, then combine this with healthy foods to come up with a meal that will make you feel content and happy for the rest of the day.

The Benefits of OMAD

When people hear about the OMAD diet, they often feel shocked. Imagine eating only one meal a day, then surviving on water and non-caloric beverages for the other 23 hours. For most people, this is too much—especially for those who are used to eating more than three times a day. But at this point, you already understand the reason behind following this diet—at least for the third week of your intuitive fasting program. There are also people who follow OMAD as part of their lifestyle. The proponents of this intense diet claim that OMAD has improved their health in so many ways.

- **Weight Loss and Fat-Burning**

As mentioned in the last section, weight loss is one of the most common benefits of the OMAD diet. This is actually a natural benefit, because you will be reducing your caloric intake each day. After a few hours of fasting, when your body is already done breaking down the food you have eaten, it will transform into a fat-burning machine. This, in turn, could add to your weight loss.

- **Increased Productivity and Freedom From Diets**

It's quite common to feel sleepy and sluggish right after lunch, especially after having a heavy meal. This could make you less productive, especially when you're at work. But if you follow OMAD and you eat your meal early in the day, you won't end up feeling this way at those times. This means that you can continue being productive while keeping yourself hydrated. Following this diet also simplifies your life, since you will only have to worry about one meal a day. This is very different from diets that come with so many strict rules and guidelines to follow.

- **Saves Time**

You will also save a lot of time when following this diet, since you only have to prepare one meal each day. After this, you can focus on doing everything else you need to do at home, at work, and even as part of your self-care routine.

- **You Will Feel More Alert Throughout the Day**

Fasting during the day causes your body to release more orexin-A. This is a type of chemical that makes you feel alert. Since you will be fasting for 23 out of 24 hours, you will definitely feel more alert throughout the day.

- **Improves the Health of Your Skin**

You have already learned all of the benefits of the different IF methods. In general, fasting improves your overall health, and that includes the health of your skin. Another surprising benefit you may notice is that you will get clearer, more supple skin as you follow this diet. This will become even more evident if you choose nourishing foods for your meals.

- **Reduced Bloating**

Bloating is another issue you may experience if you eat too much or you eat too many times throughout the day. This is another issue that you won't have to deal with on OMAD, since your body will only work to digest one meal, then take a break for the rest of the day.

- **Improved Sleep**

If you don't experience bloating, you will be able to sleep better when bedtime comes around. You can even regulate your circadian rhythm more if you eat your one meal of the day at the same time each day, preferably not right before bedtime.

These are some of the most significant benefits of the OMAD diet, and these should be enough to motivate you to stick with the diet even though it seems overwhelming. Plus, you only have to do it for a week. After this, you will give your body time to recover in the last week of the program.

Are There Any Risks?

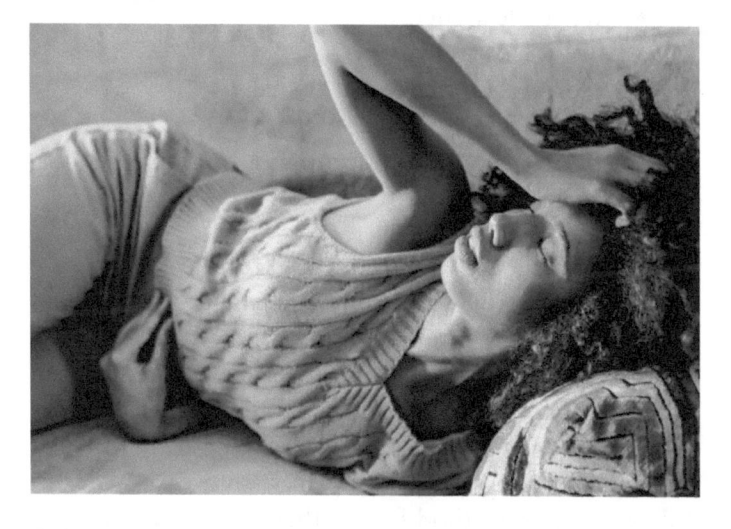

Being an intense method of fasting, OMAD does come with some risks and precautions. It's important to know these risks. too. so that you can keep an eye out for any adverse reactions you might have once you start following this IF method. Even though it's part of your intuitive fasting program, you shouldn't force yourself to endure the diet for a whole week if it's beginning to make you sick. Some of the common risks to look out for are:

- feeling extremely hungry

- binge eating when it's time to eat your meal, then feeling sick afterward

- an increase in cholesterol and blood pressure levels

- having low energy

- feeling fatigued, weak, or shaky

- having trouble concentrating or experiencing brain fog

If you start feeling any of these effects, you can ease back into your 16:8 diet. Remember that the other half of this program is intuitive eating, where you learn how to listen to your body. This is especially important when you are following OMAD, as you might feel these effects. It might be a sign that you aren't ready for such an intense fasting method yet. In such a case, you can follow the 16:8 method for another week before you try following OMAD again.

Also, if you suffer from diabetes or any other chronic medical condition, you should consult with your doctor first before you start OMAD. In fact, you should speak to your doctor first even before you start your intuitive eating program. Have a discussion about your plan for the whole four weeks, then ask your doctor how you can stay healthy throughout the program. Your doctor will probably give you the same advice about focusing on nutritious foods along with specific advice about your condition.

Conclusion

Whenever you feel challenged while following this diet (or at any other point in the program), you can motivate yourself by thinking of the goals you are trying to achieve. Also, you can go online and read about intuitive fasting success stories so that you can see how this amazing program has changed the lives of those who have followed it all the way to the end.

As you know, I am one of those people who has found success on this diet. Now, let me share with you two stories from people I personally know. I had a client named Tyler who woke up one day and decided to change his life. When he came to me, he talked about how he was tired of being pitied, belittled, and ridiculed. He was also tired of feeling so unfit and unhealthy. So, I suggested intuitive fasting to Tyler. I helped him get through the whole program, and he struggled the most during his third week. But thankfully, he stuck with the program. When he finished the 4 weeks, he had already gotten used to fasting, so he decided to continue following the 16:8 method. Around 14 months later, Tyler came to me and he looked like a different person! He lost 160 pounds and he never felt happier in his life.

Another one of my favorite success stories is from a friend-turned-client. Her name is Gigi and she lost a whopping 52 pounds in just seven months. At first, she felt skeptical. But when I shared my own journey with her, she decided to give it a try. When she started experiencing the benefits of fasting, she decided to keep going. Now, she is very happy with making healthy food choices while still being able to indulge in her cravings once in a while.

These success stories always make me feel inspired and motivated. Hopefully, they will do the same for you. Stick with the OMAD diet for seven days, and when you're done, you can give your body a break by going back to the beginning as you transition back to the 12:12 fasting method.

Chapter 9:

Phase 4: Reset and Recover

As you finish the last few days of your third week on the program, you can start planning for the fourth week. It may come as a relief to know that for the fourth week, you will be going back to the 12:12 fasting method. There is a very important reason for this, which you will discover in this chapter. Although this is the last week of your intuitive fasting program, you should still continue with all of the healthy habits you have learned thus far so that you can continue to lose weight and improve your health. But before that, you will learn the following in the sections ahead:

- Why Go Back to the 12:12 Diet?

- Healthy Lifestyle Tips

- Ways to Reduce Inflammation

Take a deep breath as you enter your final week and discover what it truly means to become a happier and healthier version of yourself.

Why Go Back to the 12:12 Fasting Method?

When you reach your fourth and final week of intuitive fasting, you will go back to following the 12:12 fasting method. The reason for changing up your eating and fasting routine is to train your metabolism to reset and recalibrate. In other words, you will keep your metabolism "on its toes."

The reason why you would go back to the 12:12 fasting method is that it takes your body up to 12 hours to use up all of the glucose from your last meal and the stored glucose in your liver. Only then will a metabolic shift happen within your body, wherein it will start utilizing your fat stores for fuel. The difference between the first week and this last week is that you should try to consume around 550 calories less than what you had been eating during the first week. Try to do this, but don't force yourself into it. Below are the benefits of going back to the 12:12 fasting method:

- **Promotes Detoxification**

Your body detoxifies itself naturally. This is a natural bodily process, just like digestion. Since fasting gives your digestive system a break, it can focus more on using its energy to eliminate toxins.

- **Reduces Inflammation**

Fasting activates the NRF2 gene pathway, which helps increase detoxification and antioxidant protection. These processes lead to a reduction in inflammation, which is a very significant benefit since inflammation is a significant factor in the development of chronic diseases.

- **Enhanced Workouts**

When you exercise while fasting, this stimulates your muscle cells to release energy through fat oxidation. This is because your glucose stores would have been depleted since you aren't eating throughout the day. In other words, exercising while you are fasting can improve your body's ability to burn fat for fuel. Fat is an excellent fuel source, and you will even notice that your strength, endurance, and energy levels increase to improve your workouts.

- **Lengthens Your Life**

This benefit comes from autophagy, one of the processes that happens during ketosis. Autophagy is a process that helps your body get rid of dead and damaged cells in order to produce new ones. This helps delay the common signs of aging and even extends your life. Many studies have shown that caloric restriction improves longevity. Fasting also stimulates the same mechanisms that prolong life by keeping calories restricted.

You may have noticed that most of the benefits offered by the different methods you will follow for each week of intuitive fasting all contribute to disease resistance. Another reason for this is that your cells experience mild stress when you are fasting. This is a healthy type of stress, as your cells learn to adapt by enhancing their ability to cope with the stress they're experiencing. This, in turn, strengthens their ability to resist disease, too.

Intuitive fasting is a four-week program that aims to put your body through varying stages and levels of stress in order to achieve weight loss. In the first week, you will incorporate fasting slowly. In the second week, you will increase your fasting window to increase the level of stress your cells feel. In the third week, you will take things even further, as you will only eat one meal per day. And in this fourth week, you will go back to the 12:12 fasting method to give your body a chance to recover, while still reaping the many benefits of the mild stress caused by fasting for 12 hours.

Now that you have gone back to the 'easier' part of your intuitive fasting program and your body has already adjusted to fasting, you can enhance the benefits even further by focusing on intuitive and mindful eating whenever you can.

Healthy Lifestyle Tips

This last week of your intuitive fasting program should also be the time when you start adapting and practicing long-term healthy habits. Remember that your goal isn't just to follow a four-week program to lose weight, then go back to your usual diet and unhealthy habits. Doing this might cause you to regain all of the weight you have lost, and everything you endured throughout the program would go to waste. To make sure that you come out of the program as a happier and healthier person, practice these healthy habits:

- **Reduce Your Consumption of Sugary Drinks**

Fruit juices, sweetened teas, sodas, and other sugary drinks are all readily available no matter where you look. But these beverages aren't good for you. They usually contain artificial and unhealthy ingredients that could increase your risk of developing type-2 diabetes, heart disease, and other conditions. If you can, stick with water and other healthy beverages.

- **Enjoy a Cup of Coffee... You Don't Have to Fear This Beverage!**

Speaking of healthy beverages, you can opt for coffee, preferably plain coffee. This is a very healthy beverage that offers loads of health benefits. Coffee is high in antioxidants, which provide protective benefits.

Drinking this in moderation is key to reaping all the benefits, though, since drinking too much might cause adverse effects like heart palpitations and sleeping issues.

- **Stay Hydrated Every Day**

This is one tip that has been stated over and over again, because you cannot disregard its importance. Even after you finish your intuitive fasting program and you start creating a plan for how to live your life in a more healthy way, staying hydrated should be part of your plan. Hydration is key to a strong and healthy body!

- **Reduce Your Sugar Intake**

Aside from sugary beverages, you should also try to limit your sugar intake altogether. Sugar can be highly addictive and, sadly, it increases your risk of various adverse conditions. This doesn't mean that you should eliminate sweets completely, though—instead, opt for more natural sources like honey, fruits, berries, or even sweeteners like stevia.

- **Avoid Foods That Are Ultra-Processed**

Just like sugary foods and beverages, ultra-processed foods aren't recommended either since they have undergone different processes that make them significantly different from their original forms. Such foods contain unhealthy ingredients like preservatives, refined sugar, refined oil, artificial coloring, and other ingredients that won't do anything good for your health. It's better to focus on whole foods that will make you feel satisfied, while also contributing to the good changes that are happening inside your body through the healthy habits you are following.

- **Eat Lots of Fruits and Vegetables**

Try to eat fruits and vegetables at every meal. These are the most nutritious foods on the planet and eating them regularly will help ensure your health. Fruits and vegetables are rich in fiber and nutrients, which your body needs to stay healthy while preventing you from eating unnecessarily throughout the day.

- **Eat Enough Protein**

Protein is also crucial for optimal health, as this macronutrient serves as raw material for building new tissues and cells. You need to eat enough protein to maintain a healthy weight without risking muscle loss. Try focusing on lean protein sources to make sure that you get all the benefits of this essential nutrient.

- **Flavor Your Meals With Herbs and Spices**

Adding herbs and spices to your dishes will make them more flavorful, while also making them more nutritious. The great thing about herbs and spices is that they are very cheap. You can even grow them at home because they are easy to grow! Instead of adding too much salt or artificial seasonings to your dishes, opt for herbs and spices instead.

- **Continue Your Active Lifestyle**

If you remember, exercising or simply adding some physical activity to your day can help you lose weight and achieve your health goals. Even after your program, you should continue your active lifestyle so that it becomes part of your life. If you can add more activities to your daily routine, that would be even better.

- **Get Enough Sleep Each Night**

When you sleep, your body is able to replenish, repair, and rejuvenate itself. If you don't get enough sleep each night, this might cause disruptions in the hormones that control your appetite, which would then cause you to struggle when you're fasting. Therefore, it's especially important to get enough sleep throughout your intuitive eating program so that you don't experience these adverse effects. Not getting enough sleep can also negatively affect your mental and physical appearance.

As you may have noticed, you can apply these healthy habits throughout your intuitive fasting program. You can even carry them over until you are done with your four weeks of intuitive fasting. I have shared these particular tips with you because they are based on scientific facts. Although these are just suggestions for you, they can help you stay healthy in the long run.

Ways to Reduce Inflammation

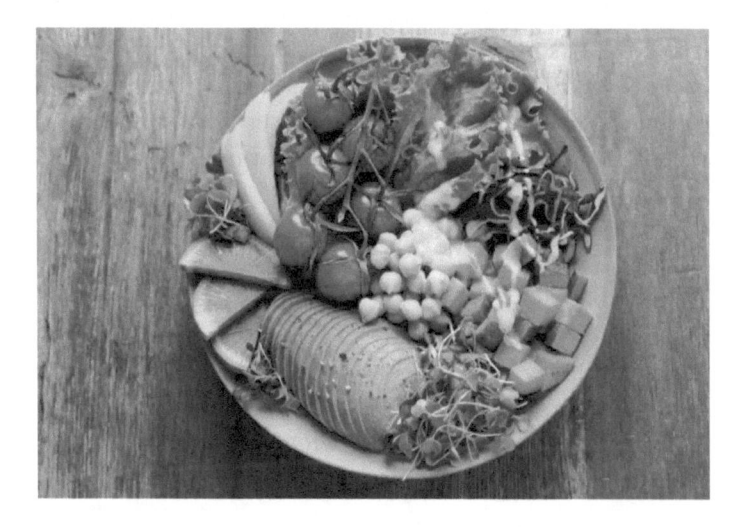

One of the most significant benefits of fasting is the reduction of inflammation. This is very important, because chronic inflammation can do a lot of damage to your body. Fasting can help manage inflammation in your body, but this isn't the only way to do so. Avoiding inflammation is another important aspect of long-term health, so let's go through some tips for how to reduce inflammation.

- **Add Anti-Inflammatory Foods to Your Diet**

Food choices are very important, whether you are fasting or you want to ensure your long-term health. While you don't have to restrict yourself from eating certain foods, it's better to focus more on nourishing your body—especially if you want to reduce inflammation. Some examples of anti-inflammatory foods that belong to your diet include fruits, vegetables, fatty fish like tuna and salmon, walnuts, soybeans, tofu, olive oil, herbs, and spices. You should also try to limit your intake of foods that cause inflammation like refined carbs, refined sugar, processed foods, red meat, deep-fried foods, corn oil, and margarine.

- **Keep Your Blood Sugar Under Control**

When your blood sugar levels fluctuate often, this could contribute to inflammation. While fasting can already help control your blood sugar levels, limiting the consumption of simple carbohydrates like refined sugar, corn syrup, white rice, and white flour can be very helpful as well.

- **Learn How to Manage Your Stress**

Chronic stress can also contribute to inflammation in your body. If you feel stressed at home and at work, you need to find ways to manage your stress more effectively. Find activities that will help you relax like yoga, meditation, guided imagery, or even taking a short walk outside to clear your head. This is especially true if you are faced with situations that you don't have control over. In such cases, you have to learn how to shift your perception, calm yourself down, and face challenges with a clear head.

- **Exercise Regularly to Lose Weight**

Exercise and physical activity can also prevent and reduce inflammation. Losing weight is also recommended. Fortunately, weight loss is one of the many benefits of intuitive fasting. If you can incorporate regular exercise into your routine as well, this will enhance the weight loss and anti-inflammatory benefits of fasting and your other healthy habits.

Reducing inflammation is essential for your health. By following these tips and all the other healthy habits you have learned so far, you can say goodbye to inflammation and all the adverse effects that come with it.

Conclusion

By the end of the fourth week, you should already start feeling the good effects of the intuitive fasting program. Now, it's time for you to continue your healthy habits to lose weight and improve your overall health long-term. After the four-week program, you can also decide which fasting method to follow. You can even switch things up every two weeks or so to reset your metabolism and ensure that your body works the way you want it to.

The intuitive fasting program is meant to help you adjust to fasting by putting your cells through varying levels of stress. And when you're done, you can keep going—but this time, you can come up with your own plan for how to continue. Before we wrap things up, one thing you should know is that at some point, you might experience some issues while fasting. These issues might cause you to feel overwhelmed to the point of giving up. But if you know what to do to overcome these issues, you can keep yourself motivated throughout the program and beyond.

Chapter 10:

Strategies for Overcoming Common Fasting Challenges

Fasting is very beneficial, but it is not the easiest thing to do—especially if you have never tried fasting before. You can experience things like extreme hunger, headaches, digestive issues, and more. Experiencing any of these adverse effects can have a negative effect on your motivation, too. But the good news is, there are ways to overcome these issues. In this chapter, we will discuss the following sections:

- People Who Shouldn't Fast

- Nine Potential Side Effects and How to Prevent or Deal With Them

Although I am a strong advocate of intuitive fasting, I want you to know both sides of the story. It's easy to claim that this is the perfect diet that will help you lose weight without feeling bad about yourself. But if you aren't aware of the potential issues that could come with this program, you might reach a point where you will think that this is just like any other diet that is too difficult to follow. So I added this chapter to prepare you for what might come and how to deal with it. That way, these issues won't stop you from achieving your goals and sticking with the program all the way to the end.

People Who Shouldn't Fast

Intuitive fasting is a combination of intuitive eating and intermittent fasting. On their own, these eating patterns have their own recommendations and risks, especially in terms of people who shouldn't follow the diet. When you combine these diets together, you will create an amazing weight loss program that also offers the benefits of both eating approaches. But this doesn't mean that intuitive fasting is completely safe for everyone. If you belong to these groups of people or you suffer from these conditions, you should think twice before starting this program:

- children and pre-teens

- teenagers

- elderly adults who experience weakness often

- elderly adults who suffer from chronic medical conditions

- pregnant or breastfeeding women

- people who suffer from dementia

- people who suffer from immunodeficiencies

- people who suffer from or have a history of eating disorders

- people who have a history of post-concussive syndrome

- people who experienced some kind of traumatic brain injury

There are other conditions and situations that could make this diet unadvisable for you. To stay on the safe side, it's best to consult with your doctor first before you decide to start with intuitive fasting. By now, you should already have a good understanding of what this program is all about. With the knowledge you have, you can start a discussion with your doctor about your plans, and find out if it is safe for you to go through with it.

Since this is a very flexible program anyway, you can still apply some of the aspects of the program to your life if your doctor advises against it. Instead of following the four-week program, you can come up with your own plan by using the tips and steps you have learned here. You might have to take things slower than the rest of us, but if that extra time will help you lose weight and achieve your goals, you can still go for it!

Nine Potential Side Effects and How to Prevent or Deal With Them

Intuitive fasting is highly effective, but it is also quite challenging—especially for beginners. Fortunately, the challenges and side effects of this program are easy to prevent and overcome. To prepare you for your intuitive fasting journey, let's go through the most common side effects of fasting and how to overcome them.

Hunger and Cravings

Since you will not eat anything for extended periods of time, hunger and cravings are inevitable. If you start slow, like giving yourself one or two weeks to adjust to fasting before diving into the program, then you might not experience extreme hunger or cravings. But if you have never tried fasting before and you start with the 12:12 method right away, expect to experience a new type of hunger that you have never experienced before.

To prevent or alleviate these issues, you can try the following:

- Whenever you feel hungry, one of the best things you can do is to drink a glass of water. Drinking water will make you feel full and it will also ensure that you don't get dehydrated. It is especially important to drink water regularly throughout your fasting periods.

- To ease the hunger you feel, you can also have a cup of plain coffee or tea. During your fasting window, you aren't allowed to consume anything with calories. So you shouldn't add milk or sugar to your coffee or tea. Switching between water, coffee, tea, and sparkling water will make your fasting period more bearable.

- When you start your intuitive fasting program, you can also start a new hobby along with it. New hobbies are exciting, and engaging in them will make time fly! Find something fun to do so that you won't have to focus on your hunger too much.

- Often, the best thing you can do to forget your hunger is by finding ways to distract yourself. You can do things like gardening, engaging in household chores, or even start working on tasks that you have been putting off—whether at home or at work. You can even engage in short, intensive exercises to get your heart pumping. The busier you are, the more you will forget your hunger.

- To help yourself calm down, try meditating for a few minutes. The great thing about meditation is that there are many ways to do it, and you only need between 10 and 15 minutes for this activity.

- Spending time in nature can be very relaxing. If you feel hungry or you're craving a certain type of food, step out the door and get a breath of fresh air. This could even count as your physical activity for the day.

To ease your cravings, allow yourself to indulge once in a while during your eating window. Take note of the cravings you feel during your fasting windows so that you can satisfy those cravings when you're allowed to eat again.

Malnutrition

This is more of a potential risk than a side effect of fasting, and it's something you should avoid. Since you will be reducing your caloric intake, especially during the third week of the intuitive fasting program, you might be at risk for nutrient deficiencies or malnutrition. To avoid this, make sure to:

- Plan your daily caloric intake by also taking into account the exercise and other physical activities you do each day. If needed, you can adjust your caloric intake.

- Focus on nourishing your body with healthy foods like fruits, vegetables, whole grains, lean proteins, healthy fats, and fish oil.

- If you end up getting sick, take a break from the program to give your body time to recuperate. If your feelings of sickness don't go away, consult with your doctor right away.

If you do visit your doctor, ask them about the possibility of taking supplements to ensure that you are getting all of the nutrients your body needs. You can also ensure that you are eating the healthiest foods possible by cooking your own meals.

Dehydration

Throughout this book, we have discussed the importance of maintaining hydration for your health. Despite this, dehydration still happens to be one of the most common side effects of fasting. To motivate yourself to drink enough water throughout the day so that you can enjoy all the benefits of the intuitive fasting diet, try the following:

- Drink a glass of water when you wake up in the morning.

- If water is too plain for you, add some mint leaves, lemon slices, or cucumber slices to your water.

- Carry a water bottle with you wherever you go.

- Download a hydration app to remind you to take water breaks throughout the day.

Making sure you drink enough water is especially important during your fasting windows when you are not consuming anything else.

Digestive Issues

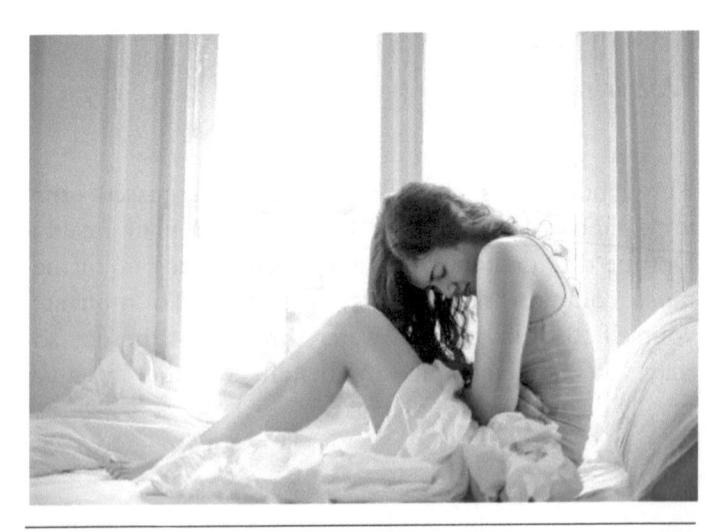

Digestive issues may come in the form of bloating, diarrhea, constipation, or nausea. You may experience these issues as your body tries to adjust to the prolonged fasting periods. Unfortunately, digestive issues could also lead to dehydration, which you should avoid. To help alleviate digestive issues while fasting, you should:

- Drink plenty of water regularly throughout the day.

- Drink electrolyte-replacement drinks or diluted juices when you're experiencing diarrhea. You can also increase your intake of foods that are high in salt and potassium.

- Consume fiber-rich foods if you are experiencing constipation.

It's also recommended to avoid sugary or highly caffeinated drinks during your eating windows if you are experiencing these issues. Following a healthy, balanced diet can also be very helpful.

Bad Breath

This is one of the more unpleasant side effects of fasting, as it can cause embarrassment—especially if someone comments on it. In this case, you can get bad breath because your mouth doesn't produce saliva as much as it should. This causes an increase in acetone, which then affects the smell of your breath. Acetone is also a by-product of fat-burning, which is why bad breath is more common when you achieve ketosis. But like any other issue that comes with fasting, there are ways to overcome this:

- Drink plenty of water to keep your mouth moist and hydrated.

- Have a proper dental hygiene routine wherein you clean all the parts of your mouth, including your tongue.

- Rinse your mouth with mouthwash after meals. You can also do this once in a while during your fasting window.

- Use breath spray or chew minty gum to mask the odor.

You can also consult with your dentist if this side effect is bothering you. Just make sure to explain that you are following a program that involves fasting so that your dentist can give you proper advice.

Headaches and Lightheadedness

Getting headaches and feeling lightheaded are also quite common when you start fasting. You may experience these during the first few days of your intuitive fasting program. There are different types of headaches and different ways to prevent or treat them:

- If you get a headache because you are dehydrated, increase your water intake. Remember that proper hydration is key throughout this program.

- If you get a headache because of caffeine withdrawal, allow yourself to have a cup of plain tea or coffee once in a while during your fasting windows. Since these are non-caloric beverages, you can drink them even while fasting.

- If you get a headache because of hypoglycemia, you need to make adjustments to your fasting routine. Either adjust your fasting and eating windows, or improve the foods you are eating during your eating windows. Limiting your carb intake for your last meal of the day can also prevent this type of headache.

If you aren't sure why you're experiencing a headache, take a break from your routine. Meditate or lie down and rest for a couple of minutes. You can also do this if you experience lightheadedness while fasting. Rest and relax to give your body time to adjust to your new routine.

Irritability and Other Mood Changes

As the days go by, you might also notice that you are more irritable than usual, and you may be experiencing other changes in your mood. This tends to happen when your blood sugar levels drop, which is a natural effect of fasting. To avoid these changes or make you feel better once you start feeling them, you can try the following:

- Again, it's important to drink water regularly. Sometimes, the 'hunger' you feel is actually your body's way of saying that you are getting dehydrated.

- When hunger strikes, brush your teeth. Simple as this activity is, it's very effective in abating your hunger.

- Drink coffee or green tea when you feel hungry, as these may help suppress your hunger.

- Keep yourself busy throughout the day. Jump from one activity to another so that you don't notice how hungry you feel.

- If you feel like you cannot stand your hunger anymore and you're about to explode, sip some bone or vegetable broth.

Also, make sure you get enough sleep each night so that you don't feel cranky and grumpy in the morning. You can also do things you really enjoy in order to lift your mood.

Fatigue and Low Energy

These are common effects, especially at the beginning of your intuitive fasting journey, since your body is still adjusting to fasting. When your blood sugar levels drop, this can cause you to have low energy levels, which then makes you feel fatigued. Some ways to avoid or overcome these issues include:

- Socializing with others—call your friends and loved ones and invite them for a cup of coffee. You can have plain coffee or tea on your date while enjoying conversations with the people closest to you. You can even suggest fun activities like going wall climbing or watching a movie.

- Play games with your family and friends. Playing and having fun releases endorphins, which will make you feel happy. This could even count as physical exercise, especially if you play games that are physically challenging.

- Sex is another enjoyable activity you can engage in, especially if you want a boost of energy.

Having sex increases your endorphins, too, which will give you a much-needed energy boost and an overall sense of well-being.

- Give aromatherapy a try. Your sense of smell is very strong, and if you smell certain scents like citrus, lavender, peppermint, and rosemary, you can feel more energized.

- Listening to music that you love can also help you overcome your low energy levels. Turn up the volume and dance along to your favorite tunes. When the song ends, find something else to do!

Sleep Issues

In some cases, people experience sleep disturbances and other sleep issues while following this program. Since getting enough sleep is essential for your success, you should overcome this issue right away. You can do this by:

- Establish a good sleep routine to help you wind down and fall asleep each night.

- Try meditation and deep breathing exercises before you sleep. You can include these in your sleep routine.

- Consider buying a memory foam mattress to make your bed more comfortable. It's also a good idea to optimize your sleeping environment so that you will feel relaxed once you go to bed.

- Go to bed earlier to give yourself more time to fall asleep. This is especially important if you need to wake up early each morning for work.

Making sure that you are well-hydrated can also help you overcome this issue. Yet another reason for you to drink water regularly—just not too close to your bedtime.

Conclusion

As I followed my own intuitive fasting program, I experienced most of the issues discussed above. The tips I shared to overcome them have worked wonders for me and they helped me succeed. One particular tip I would like to emphasize is to cook your own meals to ensure that you are eating the most nutrient-dense meals possible. Even if you don't usually cook, there are many dishes out there that you can make. I have shared some of these recipes in the next chapter for you to try out!

Chapter 11:

Sample Recipes

After understanding everything about intuitive fasting, it's time to start applying everything you have learned. To make your journey even more interesting, I would like to share with you some delicious and healthy recipes for each week of the program. In this chapter, you will learn how to make:

- Greek-Style Chickpea Waffles
- Whole Wheat Pasta With Turkey Meatballs
- Savory Fish Cakes With Dipping Sauce
- Chicken Burrito Bowls

These are just some recipe suggestions for you to try out. When I started my intuitive fasting program, these dishes were very helpful while I was fasting. They are super easy to make, they contain healthy ingredients, they are easily customizable, and eating them made me feel full and satisfied. By cooking my own meals, I was able to stick with the program for the whole four weeks. I also share recipes like these with my clients to help inspire them to cook their own food at home.

While you go through these recipes, feel free to make some changes. For instance, if you're a vegetarian, you can replace the meat with tofu or some other healthy plant-based protein source. You can use these recipes to start your intuitive fasting journey, and when you discover the joy of cooking at home, you can go online to search for more recipes!

Greek-Style Chickpea Waffles

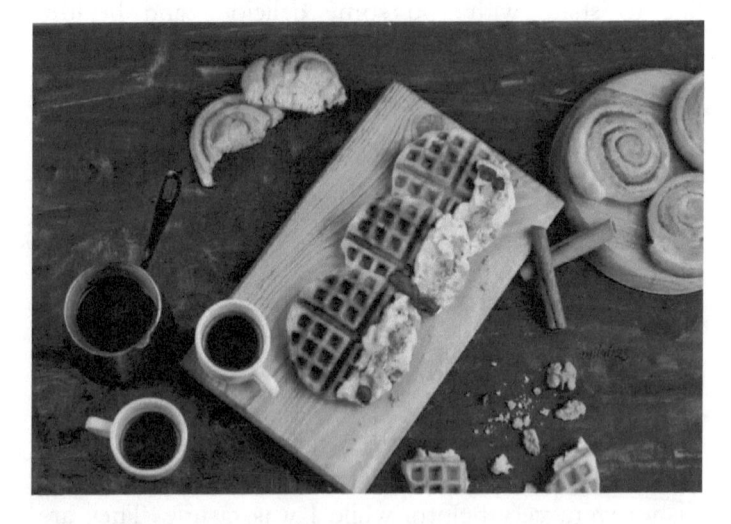

This first recipe is a wonderful example of a healthy, hearty breakfast or brunch. It's simple, delicious, and you can make it in just half an hour. While this recipe is already filling and healthy on its own, if you want it to be more filling, you can increase the protein content by adding some nuts or ham.

Time: 30 minutes
Serving Size: 2 servings
Prep Time: 10 minutes
Cook Time: 20 minutes
Ingredients:

- ½ tsp salt
- ½ tsp baking soda
- ¾ cup of 2% Greek yogurt (plain)
- ¾ cup of chickpea flour
- 6 large eggs
- Cooking spray (for cooking)
- Berries (fresh, for serving)
- Cucumber slices (for serving)
- Olive oil (for serving)
- Parsley (chopped, for serving)
- Tomatoes slices (for serving)
- Yogurt (for serving)

Directions:

1. Preheat your oven to 200°F. If needed, preheat your waffle iron as well.

2. Place a wire rack in the oven over a rimmed baking sheet.

3. In a bowl, add the chickpea flour, salt, and baking soda, then whisk well.

4. In another bowl, add the eggs and Greek yogurt, then whisk well.

5. Add the yogurt mixture into the bowl with the dry ingredients and mix until well combined.

6. Use the cooking spray to coat the preheated waffle iron.

7. Pour ¼ cup of batter into the waffle iron, close it, and cook for about 4 to 5 minutes until golden brown.

8. Transfer the cooked waffle to the baking sheet in the oven to keep it warm.

9. Repeat the cooking and warming steps until you use up all of the waffle batter.

10. Drizzle the warm waffles with olive oil and serve with cucumber slices, tomato slices, and chopped parsley for a savory meal. To make it sweet, serve the warm waffles with a dollop of yogurt and some fresh berries.

Whole Wheat Pasta With Turkey Meatballs

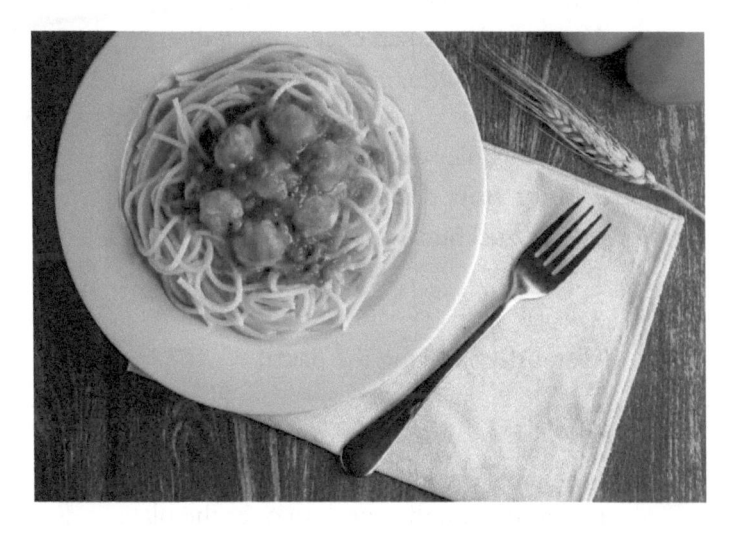

This recipe combines a hearty whole-wheat pasta with tender, juicy, and tasty meatballs to create an incredibly healthy and delicious meal. This is another simple recipe that only requires a couple of ingredients. If you want to make it even more filling and nutritious, you can add blended vegetables to the sauce before bringing everything together. This is a classic dish that will fill you up and make you feel satisfied even as you start your fasting window.

Time: 45 minutes

Serving Size: 4 servings

Prep Time: 15 minutes

Cook Time: 30 minutes

Ingredients:

- 3 tbsp olive oil
- ⅓ cup of Parmesan cheese (grated)
- 3 cups of marinara sauce (homemade or store-bought)
- 1 lb of whole-wheat pasta
- 2 lbs of ground turkey
- 1 large zucchini (chopped)
- Pepper
- Salt
- Water (for cooking the pasta)

Directions:

1. Line a plate with a few paper towels, then use a grater to grate the zucchini over the plate.

2. After grating, cover the grated zucchini with a few more paper towels, and press down to squeeze out the moisture.

3. In a bowl, add the ground turkey, Parmesan cheese, zucchini, salt, and pepper, then mix well.

4. Use your hand to take portions of the mixture, then roll each portion into a ball. Place the meatballs on a plate.

5. In a pot, add the olive oil over medium heat.

6. When the oil is hot enough, add the meatballs, and cook them until all sides are golden brown.

7. Pour the marinara sauce into the pot and mix gently.

8. Turn the heat down to low, cover the pot, and allow the mixture to simmer for about 10 to 15 minutes until the turkey meatballs are completely cooked through.

9. In a separate pot, add some water and bring to a boil.

10. Add the pasta and cook according to the directions on the packaging.

11. Once the pasta is cooked, drain the water.

12. Divide the pasta into bowls, then pour the sauce with meatballs over each serving.

13. Top with more parmesan cheese and serve with a simple side salad for a healthy, hearty meal.

Savory Fish Cakes With Dipping Sauce

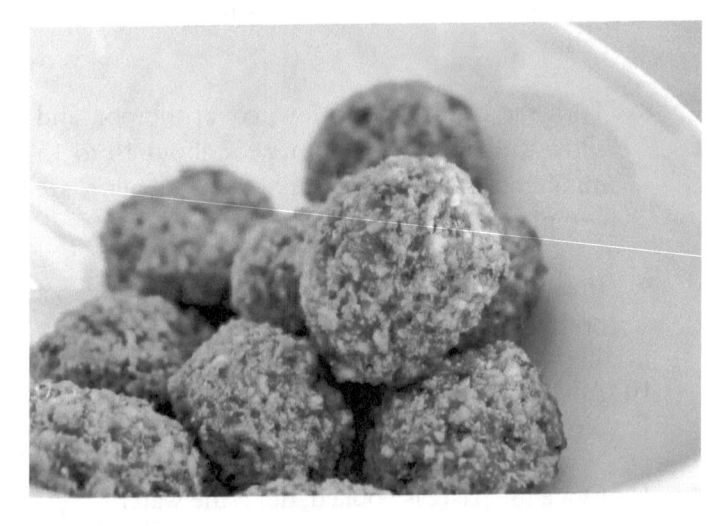

These fish cakes are the perfect low-carb appetizer, and you can even have them as a meal. This is a simple recipe that creates a healthy dish with bright flavors. It even comes with a scrumptious dipping sauce that you will surely enjoy. For this recipe, you need white fish like catfish, Pacific sole, pollock, bream, or haddock. Wild-caught fish is preferred, especially if you want to make it truly healthy. To accompany your fish cakes, you will also learn how to make a simple and refreshing mango salsa that's super easy to make, too. This mouthwatering combination will make you feel happy and satisfied after eating.

Time: 30 minutes
Serving Size: 2 servings
Prep Time: 20 minutes
Cook Time: 10 minutes
Ingredients for the fish cakes:

- 2 tbsp coconut oil
- ¼ cup of cilantro (chopped)
- 1 lb white fish (boneless)
- 2 cloves of garlic (minced)
- Chili flakes
- Salt
- Avocado oil (for greasing your hands, you can also use any neutral oil)

Ingredients for the dipping sauce:

- 2 tbsp water
- 3 tbsp lemon juice (freshly squeezed)
- 2 avocados (ripe)
- Salt

Ingredients for the mango salsa:

- ⅛ cup of lime juice (freshly squeezed)
- ⅛ cup of packed cilantro leaves (fresh, chopped)
- ¼ cup of red onion (chopped)
- 1 small jalapeño (seeded, minced)
- 1 small red bell pepper (chopped)
- 2 mangoes (ripe, diced)

- Salt

Directions:

1. In a food processor, add all of the fish cake ingredients except the avocado oil, then pulse until all of the ingredients are well combined.

2. Use avocado oil to grease your hands, then take portions of the mixture, and form them into small patties.

3. In a frying pan, add the coconut oil over medium-high heat. Swirl the pan around to coat the whole surface with the oil.

4. When the oil is hot enough, add the fish cakes.

5. Cook for about 4 to 5 minutes on each side until cooked through and golden brown on the outside.

6. Place the cooked fish cakes on a plate lined with a paper towel to drain the excess oils. Set aside.

7. Rinse the food processor, then add all of the dipping sauce ingredients. Pulse until you get a creamy and smooth texture.

8. Pour the sauce into a small bowl, then place the bowl in the middle of the plate with the fishcakes.

9. In a bowl, add the bell pepper, mango, cilantro, jalapeño, and onion, then mix well.

10. Sprinkle some salt over the salsa, drizzle with lime juice, then mix well.

11. Serve the fish cakes while warm with dipping sauce and mango salsa on the side. You can even fry some chorizo slices and add these to your dish for a protein boost and a real flavor punch!

Chicken Burrito Bowls

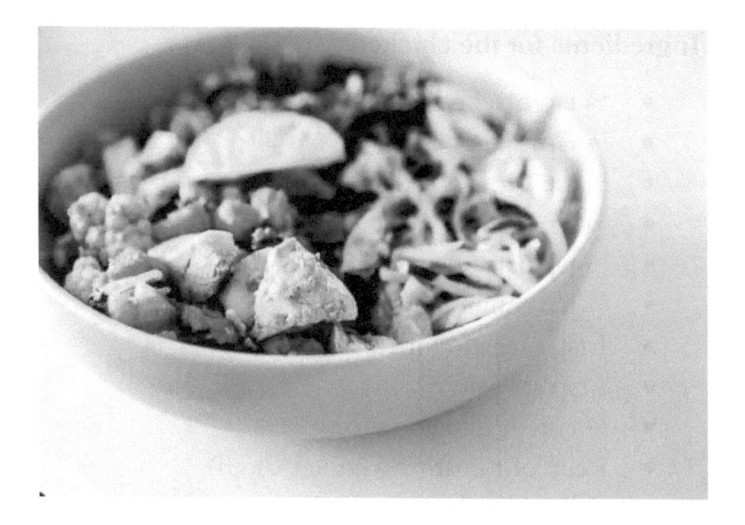

Although this dish takes a lot of time to make (mainly because you will cook the chicken in the slow cooker), it's definitely worth the time and effort. This dish is super healthy as it's made with cauliflower rice, and is also filling because of all the healthy ingredients each burrito bowl contains. To make this a vegetarian dish, substitute the chicken for tofu, tempeh, or jackfruit so you will still get protein and other essential nutrients. After following this dish, you can also try mixing up the toppings to see which combinations make you feel happy with each bite. You can even add more ingredients to this dish since it's easily customizable.

Time: 3 hours, 10 minutes

Serving Size: 3 servings

Prep Time: 10 minutes

Cook Time: 3 hours

Ingredients for the chicken:

- ⅛ tsp cayenne
- ¼ tsp chili powder
- ¼ tsp garlic powder
- ¼ tsp paprika
- ½ tsp black pepper
- ½ tsp cumin (ground)
- 1 tsp oregano (dried)
- 1 tsp sea salt
- ½ cup of tomato sauce
- 1 cup of tomatoes (canned, diced)
- ½ lb of chicken breasts (boneless, skinless)
- ½ lb of chicken thighs (boneless, skinless)
- ¼ jalapeño (seeded and diced)

- 1 small yellow onion (diced)

Ingredients for the cauliflower rice:

- ¼ tsp black pepper
- ¼ tsp garlic powder
- ¾ tsp sea salt
- ½ tbsp olive oil
- 1 head of cauliflower (cut into florets)

Ingredients for assembling the burrito bowls:

- 1 cup of black beans (canned, drained)
- 1 tomato (diced)
- 1 avocado (peeled, pitted, cut into cubes)
- Optional toppings like Greek yogurt (plain) or lime wedges

Directions:

1. In the bowl of your slow cooker, add all of the chicken ingredients.

2. Place the bowl in the slow cooker, cover with a lid, and cook the chicken for about 2 to 3 hours on high.

3. After cooking, use two forks to shred the chicken.

4. Pour some of the juices into a small bowl and set aside.

5. Mix the shredded chicken with the juices, then place it back into the slow cooker while you prepare the other ingredients.

6. In a food processor, add the cauliflower florets, then pulse until you get a rice-like consistency.

7. In a pan, add the olive oil over medium-high heat.

8. When the oil is hot enough, add the riced cauliflower, then cook for about 8 to 10 minutes.

9. Add the seasonings and mix well.

10. Divide the cooked cauliflower rice into bowls.

11. In a separate bowl, add the beans and the juices from the cooked chicken, then mix well.

12. Top each bowl with shredded chicken, beans, tomatoes, and avocado.

13. Add a dollop of Greek yogurt to each bowl, then serve immediately with lime wedges.

Conclusion

Since intuitive fasting is an extremely flexible program in terms of the foods you can eat, you have the option to choose all of the tasty, delicious, and healthy meals you want to eat when you're not fasting. In this chapter, you have learned how to make four different recipes that are filling, mouthwatering, and oh-so-easy to make. Now that you have tried cooking these simple meals, you can go online and look for more recipes to keep you satisfied while you embark on your intuitive fasting journey. The more you cook, the easier it will get. Soon, you will be wondering how you survived in the past without making your own meals!

Conclusion:

Start Your Weight Loss Journey Now!

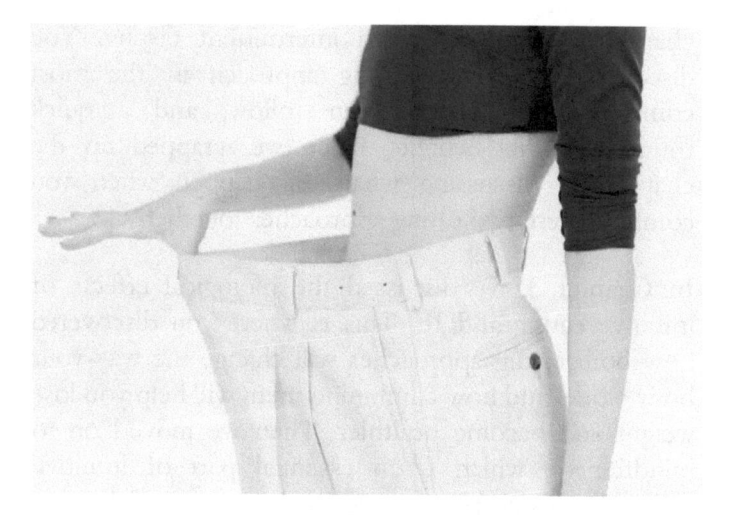

There you have it. Everything you need to know to start your own intuitive fasting journey. Throughout this book, you discovered what intuitive fasting means, and also the two eating approaches that make up this powerful weight-loss program. We started your learning journey by defining what intuitive fasting is. You learned the fundamentals of the diet, its history, and the two eating approaches that have been combined to create this program: intuitive eating and intermittent fasting.

In the next chapter, we discussed these two eating approaches separately. First, we focused on intuitive eating, what it means, and the 10 core principles that the eating approach is based on. As you have learned, intuitive fasting is all about listening to your body and awakening your inner intuition. In order to satisfy your true hunger, you need to learn how to differentiate physical hunger from emotional hunger. In the same chapter, we also discussed intermittent fasting. You discovered what this eating approach is, the most common methods you can follow, and a quick rundown of its benefits. Then we wrapped up the chapter by discussing what will happen when you combine these two eating approaches together.

In Chapter 3, we discussed the biological effects of intuitive eating and IF. This is where you discovered how both eating approaches will change the way your body works and how combining them will help you lose weight and become healthier. Then we moved on to mindfulness, which is an essential part of intuitive eating. In this chapter, you learned what mindful eating is, how to practice it, and other ways to listen to your body.

But before you start following your intuitive fasting program, you should be aware of the most important nutrients your body needs to stay healthy. So in the next chapter, we focused on supplements. We enumerated the most important vitamins and minerals, their significance to your health, where you can get those nutrients, and why you need to take supplements in case you don't get enough. In the next four chapters, we discussed the different phases of the intuitive fasting program. We broke down each phase to make it easier for you to understand what is involved, the recommended foods to eat, and the benefits of the fasting methods involved in each.

In Chapter 10, you learned about how to overcome the most common fasting challenges. The steps you learned here can help you find success as you start following the program. You can even keep coming back to this book and use it as a reference when you feel challenged at any point during your program. And in the final chapter, I shared some easy, filling, and delicious recipes with you. I made these dishes for myself while I was following the program, and they really helped me stick with each week of the program even though it became more and more challenging.

When I finished my intuitive fasting program, I discovered that I had picked up some new eating habits. These healthier eating habits allowed me to keep losing weight until I reached my target. Once that happened, I continued eating healthily to maintain my healthy weight. Now that you know a lot of tips and techniques to succeed in intuitive fasting, it's time to start applying what you have learned. As time goes by, watch those pounds melt away quicker than you think! Once you start, you will be on your way to becoming a happier, healthier you—the easy way. Hopefully, this book has motivated and inspired you to start changing your life. If you would also like to share what you have learned here so other people can improve their lives too, you can leave a review for others to read. I would really appreciate it! Good luck with your journey and I hope that by the end, you can continue to lead a healthier lifestyle, too.

Thank you for your recent purchase of this book.

I hope you love it! I'd kindly like to ask you to leave a brief review on Amazon. Reviews aren't easy to come by, but they have a profound impact. So, we would be incredibly thankful if you could just take a minute to leave a quick review, even if it's just a sentence or two!

You can do it simply just clicking this link:
https://www.amazon.com/review/create-review?asin=B0B3W6XK6C

Thank you so much for taking the time to leave a short review. We are very appreciative as your review makes a difference. This will help me keep up with your needs and also help others like you to find this helpful book. Review or not, we still love you!!

You can subscribe on my page and as a Thank you I'll give you a Free copy of my secrets of incredible weight loss e-book.

Simply subscribe by clicking this link:
www.jannahadams.com

References

Anderson, L. (2022, January 3). *Five-ingredient turkey meatballs with whole wheat pasta.* Craving California. https://cravingcalifornia.com/five-ingredient-turkey-meatballs

Anderson, L. M., Reilly, E. E., Schaumberg, K., Dmochowski, S., & Anderson, D. A. (2015). *Contributions of mindful eating, intuitive eating, and restraint to BMI, disordered eating, and meal consumption in college students.* Eating and Weight Disorders - Studies on Anorexia, Bulimia and Obesity, 21(1), 83–90. https://doi.org/10.1007/s40519-015-0210-3

Asprey, D. (2021). *Intuitive fasting, metabolic flexibility & metaphysical meals - Dr. Will Cole with Dave Asprey - #796.* Dave Asprey. https://daveasprey.com/dr-will-cole-796

Baier, L. (2018). *Slow cooker chicken burrito bowls.* A Sweet Pea Chef. https://www.asweetpeachef.com/slow-cooker-chicken-burrito-bowls

Bailey, D. L. (2017). *If you have discipline, drive and determination...nothing is impossible. -* Dana Linn Bailey. Millionaire Mindset.

https://www.millionairemindset.net/if-you-have-discipline-drive-and-determination-nothing-is-impossible-dana-linn-bailey

Berman, R. (2016, March 26). *What is your metabolic rate?*. Dummies. https://www.dummies.com/article/body-mind-spirit/physical-health-well-being/common-ailments/metabolism/what-is-your-metabolic-rate-166873

Bjarnadottir, A. (2019, February 15). *8 Foods that beat a multivitamin*. Healthline. https://www.healthline.com/nutrition/8-foods-that-beat-a-multivitamin

Byakodi, R. (2021, December 1). *12 Hour intermittent fasting: A guide on 12 hour fast*. 21 Day Hero. https://21dayhero.com/12-hour-intermittent-fasting

Chander, R. (2020, June 3). *I tried extreme fasting by eating once a day — Here's what happened*. Healthline. https://www.healthline.com/health/food-nutrition/one-meal-a-day-diet

Charles, S. (2021, February 4). *What is HGH?*. Verywell Health. https://www.verywellhealth.com/what-is-hgh-5078922

Clear, J. (2012). *The beginner's guide to intermittent fasting*. https://jamesclear.com/the-beginners-guide-to-intermittent-fasting

Collier, R. (2013). *Intermittent fasting: The science of going without.* Canadian Medical Association Journal, 185(9), E363–E364. https://doi.org/10.1503/cmaj.109-4451

Cookie and Kate. (2015). *Fresh mango salsa.* https://cookieandkate.com/fresh-mango-salsa-recipe

Cronkleton, E. (2019, March 29). *Why is Vitamin B complex important, and where do I get it?.* Healthline. https://www.healthline.com/health/food-nutrition/vitamin-b-complex#complications-tied-to-deficiency

Davis, T. (2019, July 31). *How to eat mindfully by listening to your body.* Greater Good. https://greatergood.berkeley.edu/article/item/how_to_eat_mindfully_by_listening_to_your_body

Denny, K. N., Loth, K., Eisenberg, M. E., & Neumark-Sztainer, D. (2013). *Intuitive eating in young adults. Who is doing it, and how is it related to disordered eating behaviors?.* Appetite, 60, 13–19. https://doi.org/10.1016/j.appet.2012.09.029

Devje, S. (2022, January 14). *Vitamin D benefits.* Healthline. https://www.healthline.com/health/food-nutrition/benefits-vitamin-d

Dr. Will Cole. (n.d.-a). *About Dr. Will Cole.* DrWillCole.com. https://drwillcole.com/about

Dr. Will Cole. (n.d.-b). *Intuitive fasting.* DrWillCole.com. https://drwillcole.com/intuitive-fasting

Dunkin, M. A. (2021, May 16). *Human growth hormone (HGH).* WebMD. https://www.webmd.com/fitness-exercise/human-growth-hormone-hgh#1

Editorial Staff. (2020, August 20). *The facts about fasting diets.* Tufts Health & Nutrition Letter. https://www.nutritionletter.tufts.edu/healthy-eating/the-facts-about-fasting-diets

The Editors of Women's Health. (2020, January 30). *Need an intermittent fasting meal plan? Here's your 7-Day brunch and dinner plan to break your fast.* Women's Health. https://www.womenshealthmag.com/weight-loss/a30658778/intermittent-fasting-meal-plan-men-s-health

Endocrine Society. (2022, January 23). *Pancreas hormones.* Endocrine.org. https://www.endocrine.org/patient-engagement/endocrine-library/hormones-and-endocrine-function/pancreas-hormones

Etienne-Mesubi, M. (2021, February 15). *The right way to do OMAD (One meal a day).* LIFE Apps.

https://lifeapps.io/fasting/the-right-way-to-do-omad-one-meal-a-day

Gala, T. (2022). *8 Supplements everyone should take: Feel healthier and reduce inflammation with these essential nutrients.* Drthadgala.com. https://drthadgala.com/8-supplements-everyone-should-take-feel-healthier-and-reduce-inflammation-with-these-essential-nutrients

Garone, S. (2021, June 27). *What is the difference between mindful and intuitive eating?.* Verywell Fit. https://www.verywellfit.com/what-is-the-difference-between-mindful-and-intuitive-eating-5185142

Gunnars, K. (2019, May 28). *Omega-3 fatty acids — The ultimate beginner's guide.* Healthline. https://www.healthline.com/nutrition/omega-3-guide#food-sources

Gunnars, K. (2020a, April 20). *Intermittent fasting 101 — The ultimate beginner's guide.* Healthline. https://www.healthline.com/nutrition/intermittent-fasting-guide#_noHeaderPrefixedContent

Gunnars, K. (2020b, December 9). *Probiotics 101: A simple beginner's guide.* Healthline. https://www.healthline.com/nutrition/probiotics-101

Gunnars, K. (2022, March 10). 27 *Health and nutrition tips that are actually evidence-based.* Healthline.

https://www.healthline.com/nutrition/27-health-and-nutrition-tips

Hazzard, V. M., Telke, S. E., Simone, M., Anderson, L. M., Larson, N. I., & Neumark-Sztainer, D. (2020). *Intuitive eating longitudinally predicts better psychological health and lower use of disordered eating behaviors: Findings from EAT 2010–2018.* Eating and Weight Disorders - Studies on Anorexia, Bulimia and Obesity. https://doi.org/10.1007/s40519-020-00852-4

Helpguide. (2019). *Vitamins and minerals.* HelpGuide.org https://www.helpguide.org/harvard/vitamins-and-minerals.htm

Hess-Fischl, A., & Jaffe, L. (2021, July 15). *What is insulin?.* EndocrineWeb. https://www.endocrineweb.com/conditions/type-1-diabetes/what-insulin

Intuitive Eating. (n.d.). *10 Principles of intuitive eating.* IntuitiveEating.org. https://www.intuitiveeating.org/10-principles-of-intuitive-eating

Jarreau, P. (2019, April 15). *How to practice intermittent fasting safely.* LIFE Apps. https://lifeapps.io/fasting/how-to-practice-intermittent-fasting-safely

Jennings, K.-A. (2019, June 25). *A quick guide to intuitive eating.* Healthline.

https://www.healthline.com/nutrition/quick-guide-intuitive-eating

Jerath, R., Edry, J. W., Barnes, V. A., & Jerath, V. (2006). *Physiology of long pranayamic breathing: Neural respiratory elements may provide a mechanism that explains how slow deep breathing shifts the autonomic nervous system.* Medical Hypotheses, 67(3), 566–571. https://doi.org/10.1016/j.mehy.2006.02.042

Joe. (2022). *The golden rules of intuitive eating and intutaive fasting.* 9 to 5 Nutrition. https://9-to-5-nutrition.com/intuitive-eating-intutaive-fasting

John Hopkins Medicine. (2021). *Intermittent fasting: What is it, and how does it work?.* https://www.hopkinsmedicine.org/health/wellness-and-prevention/intermittent-fasting-what-is-it-and-how-does-it-work

Kaupe, A. (2021a, December 1). *Intermittent fasting headache: Here's how to cure it.* 21 Day Hero. https://21dayhero.com/intermittent-fasting-headache

Kaupe, A. (2021b, December 1). *OMAD results: What to expect from one meal a day diet.* 21 Day Hero. https://21dayhero.com/omad-results

Kerin, J. L., Webb, H. J., & Zimmer-Gembeck, M. J. (2019). *Intuitive, mindful, emotional, external and regulatory eating behaviours and beliefs: An investigation of the core components.* Appetite, 132, 139–146. https://doi.org/10.1016/j.appet.2018.10.011

Landsverk, G. (2021, March 5). *Gwyneth Paltrow is using an 'intuitive fasting' diet to treat lingering COVID-19 symptoms.* Insider. https://www.insider.com/gwyneth-paltrow-intuitive-fasting-to-treat-symptoms-of-covid-19-2021-3

Leeds, W. (2019). *How to listen to your body and give it what it needs.* Tiny Buddha. https://tinybuddha.com/blog/how-listen-to-your-body-and-give-it-what-it-needs

Leonard, J. (2020, January 17). *A guide to 16:8 intermittent fasting.* Medical News Today. https://www.medicalnewstoday.com/articles/327398

Lindberg, S. (2018, August 23). *Autophagy: What you need to know.* Healthline. https://www.healthline.com/health/autophagy

London, J. (2019, May 28). *What is the OMAD Diet? What you need to know about this intermittent fasting weight-loss plan.* Good Housekeeping. https://www.goodhousekeeping.com/health/diet-nutrition/a27506052/omad-diet

London, J. (2020, July 14). *What you should know about the 16:8 diet before you start fasting.* Good

Housekeeping. https://www.goodhousekeeping.com/health/diet-nutrition/a27336892/16-8-diet

Longo, V. D., & Mattson, M. P. (2014). *Fasting: Molecular mechanisms and clinical applications.* Cell Metabolism, 19(2), 181–192. https://doi.org/10.1016/j.cmet.2013.12.008

Martin, B., Mattson, M. P., & Maudsley, S. (2006). *Caloric restriction and intermittent fasting: Two potential diets for successful brain aging.* Ageing Research Reviews, 5(3), 332–353. https://doi.org/10.1016/j.arr.2006.04.002

McAuliffe, L. (2022, January 3). *16/8 Intermittent fasting: Benefits and tips for getting started.* Dr. Robert Kiltz. https://www.doctorkiltz.com/16-8-intermittent-fasting

Meier, M. (2021, April 21). *What is intuitive fasting and why does Gwyneth Paltrow do it?.* BodyandSoul.com.au. https://www.bodyandsoul.com.au/nutrition/what-is-intuitive-fasting-and-why-does-gwyneth-paltrow-do-it/news-story/b770d8fbb111c6c5d8837681c1e6cdd5

MindFood. (2020, September 10). *The top 10 most addictive foods, according to science.* MindFood.com. https://www.mindfood.com/article/the-hardest-foods-to-stop-eating

Palsdottir, H. (2021, January 28). *Do multivitamins work? The surprising truth.* Healthline. https://www.healthline.com/nutrition/do-multivitamins-work

Paltrow, G. (2021, February 11). *Gwyneth on Intuitive Fasting.* Goop. https://goop.com/wellness/health/gwyneth-paltrow-on-intuitive-fasting

Petersen, K. S. (n.d.). *Intuitive fasting: Why this "third way" of living could be better.* Inverse. https://www.inverse.com/mind-body/intuitive-fasting

Petrucci, K., & Flynn, P. (2016, March 27). *10 Ways to feel energized when you're fasting.* Dummies. https://www.dummies.com/article/body-mind-spirit/physical-health-well-being/diet-nutrition/general-diet-nutrition/10-ways-to-feel-energized-when-youre-fasting-203867

Petrucci, K., & Flynn, P. (2017, April 11). *9 Ways to stave off hunger when fasting.* Dummies. https://www.dummies.com/article/body-mind-spirit/physical-health-well-being/diet-nutrition/general-diet-nutrition/9-ways-to-stave-off-hunger-when-fasting-203866

Pie, J. (2018, July 31). *Keto fish cakes with avocado lemon dipping sauce.* Bulletproof. https://www.bulletproof.com/recipes/eating-healthy/fish-cakes-recipe-2g

Pike, A. (2020, June 19). *The science behind intuitive eating.* Food Insight. https://foodinsight.org/the-science-behind-intuitive-eating

Price, C. J., & Hooven, C. (2018). *Interoceptive awareness skills for emotion regulation: Theory and approach of mindful awareness in body-oriented therapy (MABT).* Frontiers in Psychology, 9. https://doi.org/10.3389/fpsyg.2018.00798

Pridgett, T. (2018, October 1). *I fasted 12 hours for 21 days — Here are the 3 Major changes that happened to my body.* POPSUGAR Fitness UK. https://www.popsugar.co.uk/fitness/What-1212-Fasting-45330857?utm_medium=redirect&utm_campaign=US:DK&utm_source=www.google.com

Schnurbusch, E. (2019, March 8). *7 Tips for staying hydrated.* Sentara. https://www.sentara.com/healthwellness/data/blogs/7-tips-for-staying-hydrated.aspx

Schram, A. E. (2022, January 12). *The beginner's guide to intuitive eating.* Kara Lydon. https://karalydon.com/health-wellness/beginners-guide-intuitive-eating

Scripps Health. (2020, January 15). *Six keys to reducing inflammation.* Scripps.org. https://www.scripps.org/news_items/4232-six-keys-to-reducing-inflammation

Segal, J., Robinson, L., & Cruz, M. (2020). *Mindful eating.* Help Guide. https://www.helpguide.org/articles/diets/mindful-eating.htm

Snyder, A. (2019, October 7). *Diarrhea during fasting and other side effects.* Healthline. https://www.healthline.com/health/diarrhea-during-fasting

Southard, L. (2022, January 28). *What is the OMAD diet? Why eating one meal a day isn't recommended by dietitians.* Insider. https://www.insider.com/omad-diet

Sreenivas, S. (2021, March 5). *What is intuitive eating?.* WebMD. https://www.webmd.com/diet/what-is-intuitive-eating#1

Streit, L., & Link, R. (2021, December 17). *What is 16/8 intermittent fasting? A beginner's guide.* Healthline. https://www.healthline.com/nutrition/16-8-intermittent-fasting

Susarla Primary Care. (2019, July 3). *How to prevent getting HANGRY during fasting?.* https://susarlapc.com/how-to-prevent-getting-hangry-during-fasting

Tabalia, J. (2020, October 23). *12-Hour intermittent fasting for weight loss and other benefits.* BetterMe Blog. https://betterme.world/articles/12-hour-intermittent-fasting

The iDiet. (2016). *The science of weight loss.* https://www.theidiet.com/science-weight-loss

Tinsley, G. (2021, April 23). *9 Potential intermittent fasting side effects.* Healthline. https://www.healthline.com/nutrition/intermittent-fasting-side-effects

Tribole, E. (2019, July 17). *Definition of intuitive eating.* Intuitive Eating. https://www.intuitiveeating.org/definition-of-intuitive-eating

Tunstall, R. J., Mehan, K. A., Hargreaves, M., Spriet, L. L., & Cameron-Smith, D. (2002). *Fasting activates the gene expression of UCP3 independent of genes necessary for lipid transport and oxidation in skeletal muscle.* Biochemical and Biophysical Research Communications, 294(2), 301–308. https://doi.org/10.1016/S0006-291X(02)00473-4

U.S. National Heart, Lung, and Blood Institute. (2019). *Calculate your BMI - standard BMI calculator.* Nih.gov. https://www.nhlbi.nih.gov/health/educational/lose_wt/BMI/bmicalc.htm

U.S. National Institutes of Health. (2021, March 26). *Vitamin C.* Nih.gov. https://ods.od.nih.gov/factsheets/VitaminC-HealthProfessional

U.S. National Institutes of Health. (2021, August 4). *Omega-3 fatty acids*. Nih.gov. https://ods.od.nih.gov/factsheets/Omega3FattyAcids-Consumer

UltraDEX. (n.d.). *Hunger breath: What causes it and how to get rid of it*. Ultradex.co.uk. https://ultradex.co.uk/hunger-breath-what-causes-it-and-how-to-get-rid-of-it

Van Dyke, N., & Drinkwater, E. J. (2013). *Review article relationships between intuitive eating and health indicators:* Literature review. Public Health Nutrition, 17(8), 1757–1766. https://doi.org/10.1017/s1368980013002139

Wakefit Team. (2020, March 2). *Effects of fasting on sleep*. Wakefit. https://www.wakefit.co/blog/effects-fasting-sleep

Ware, M. (2020, January 6). *Why do we need magnesium?*. Medical News Today. https://www.medicalnewstoday.com/articles/286839

Warren, J. M., Smith, N., & Ashwell, M. (2017). *A structured literature review on the role of mindfulness, mindful eating and intuitive eating in changing eating behaviours: Effectiveness and associated potential mechanisms*. Nutrition Research Reviews, 30(2), 272–283. https://doi.org/10.1017/s0954422417000154

WebMD. (2021a, May 18). *Why you need zinc and how to get it.* WebMD.com. https://www.webmd.com/diet/ss/slideshow-zinc-mineral

WebMD. (2021b, May 20). *Risks and benefits of probiotics.* WebMD.com. https://www.webmd.com/digestive-disorders/probiotics-risks-benefits

WebMD Editorial Contributors. (2021, April 8). *Is eating one meal a day safe?.* WebMD. https://www.webmd.com/diet/is-eating-one-meal-a-day-safe#1

Weiss, C. (n.d.). *Statistics on Dieting and Eating Disorders.* Montenido.com. https://www.montenido.com/pdf/montenido_statistics.pdf

Zauner, C., Schneeweiss, B., Kranz, A., Madl, C., Ratheiser, K., Kramer, L., Roth, E., Schneider, B., & Lenz, K. (2000). *Resting energy expenditure in short-term starvation is increased as a result of an increase in serum norepinephrine.* The American Journal of Clinical Nutrition, 71(6), 1511–5. https://doi.org/10.1093/ajcn/71.6.1511

Zelman, K. M. (2020, September 12). *The benefits of Vitamin C.* WebMD. https://www.webmd.com/diet/features/the-benefits-of-vitamin-c#1

Zhu, Y., Yan, Y., Gius, D. R., & Vassilopoulos, A. (2013). *Metabolic regulation of Sirtuins upon fasting and the implication for cancer.* Current Opinion in Oncology, 25(6), 630–636. https://doi.org/10.1097/01.cco.0000432527.49984.a3

Image References

Castillo, L. (2021). *White ceramic bowl with noodle and chicken*. Pexels. [Image]. https://www.pexels.com/photo/white-ceramic-bowl-with-noodle-and-chicken-9213869

Gianyasa. (2021). *[Spaghetti and meatballs]*. Pixabay. [Image]. https://pixabay.com/photos/spaghetti-spaghetti-and-meatballs-6681830

Grabowska, K. (2020a). *Wake up and workout title on light box surface surrounded by colorful sport equipment*. Pexels. [Image]. https://www.pexels.com/photo/wake-up-and-workout-title-on-light-box-surface-surrounded-by-colorful-sport-equipment-4397841

Grabowska, K. (2020b). *Woman in loose denim measuring her waistline*. Pexels. [Image]. https://www.pexels.com/photo/woman-in-loose-denim-measuring-her-waistline-5714344

Klavins, R. (2021). *Capsules pill and drug sig*. Unsplash. [Image]. https://unsplash.com/photos/n-7HTOiJPso

Krivec, A. (2014). *Roman numerals on alarm clock.* Unsplash. [Image]. https://unsplash.com/photos/ZMZHcvIVgbg

Olsson, E. (2019). *Salmon and quinoa dish.* Unsplash. [Image]. https://unsplash.com/photos/KPDbRyFOTnE

Pelzer, A. (2017). *Vegan salad bowl.* Unsplash. [Image]. https://unsplash.com/photos/IGfIGP5ONV0

Piacquadio, A. (2018a). *Photo of woman looking at the mirror.* Pexels. [Image]. https://www.pexels.com/photo/photo-of-woman-looking-at-the-mirror-774866

Piacquadio, A. (2018b). *Woman suffering from a stomach pain.* Pexels. [Image]. https://www.pexels.com/photo/woman-suffering-from-a-stomach-pain-3807756

Shimazaki, S. (2020). *Black woman having head ache.* Pexels. [Image]. https://www.pexels.com/photo/black-woman-having-head-ache-5938367

SHVETS production. (2021). *Crop woman in oversized pants.* Pexels. [Image]. https://www.pexels.com/photo/crop-woman-in-oversized-pants-6975481

Uniqueton, A. (2020). *Breaded shrimps in rice balls in close up photography*. Pexels. [Image]. https://www.pexels.com/photo/breaded-shrimps-in-rice-balls-in-close-up-photography-4722522

White, B. (2016). *Contemplating woman*. Unsplash. [Image]. https://unsplash.com/photos/qYanN54gIrI

Zahedi, B. (2020). *Coffee, waffles and cinnamon rolls*. Pexels. [Image]. https://www.pexels.com/photo/coffee-waffles-and-cinnamon-rolls-5253075

Zuzyusa. (2018). Weight Loss. Pixabay. [Image]. https://pixabay.com/photos/fitnessstrengthening-exercises-3167418/

Made in United States
Troutdale, OR
11/19/2023

14751915R00116